Chronicle

The
Botanical
Beauty
Hunter

To Mother Earth.
For the animals, trees and flowers, and
for reminding us we are never alone.

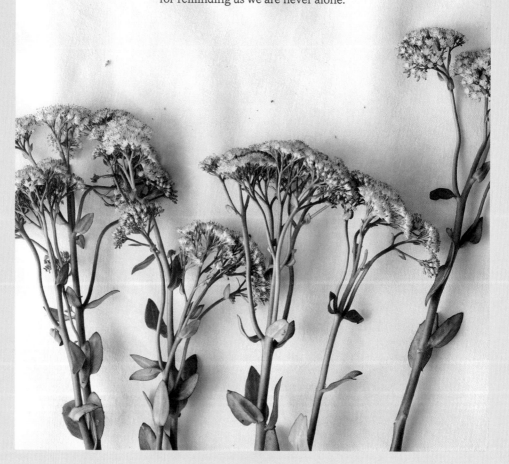

The Botanical Beauty Hunter

Natural recipes and rituals for
skincare, haircare and cosmetics

Maddy Dixon

Hardie Grant

BOOKS

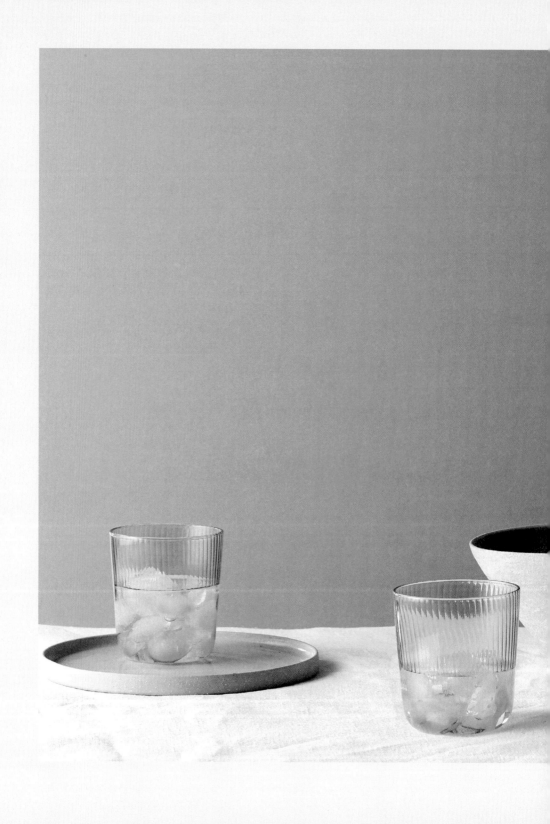

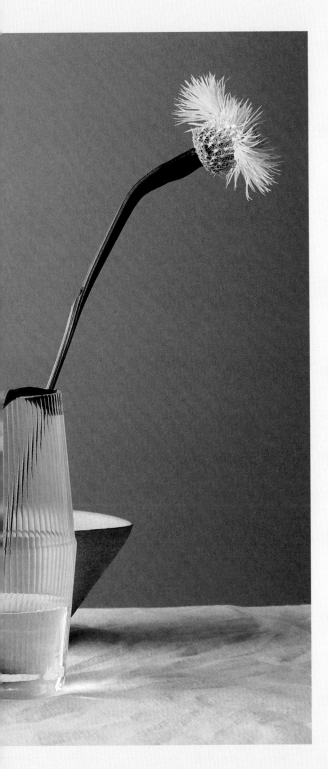

Contents

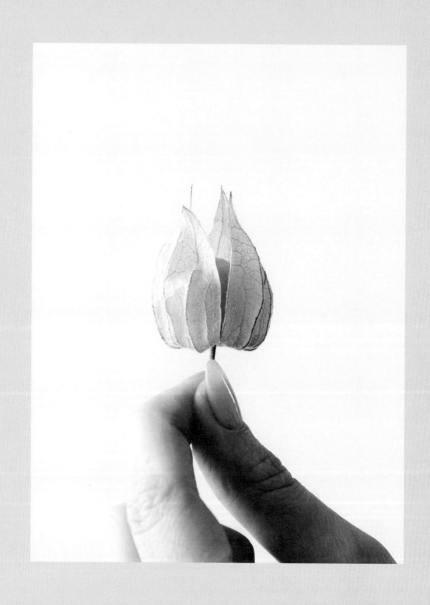

Intro

I live by the motto that beauty is wellness and wellness is beauty. It's my hobby, my passion and the thing I most love sharing with other people. From diet and meditation to acupuncture facials, if it's wellness related – I'll try it. It's important to know how to look after and care for yourself. Not just so you feel and look your most radiant, but also so you're able to be your best for those around you. Wellness suffuses all aspects of my life: from the food I eat and the thoughts I train myself to think to the beauty products and rituals I incorporate into my life. But don't be fooled – it wasn't always this way!

I worked as a model for more than ten years, travelling the world, having a fabulous time and immersing myself in the beauty industry. It all looked like everything was going along just swimmingly, but the truth is, I was struggling. I forged forward, but I knew even then that being a model was not what I was put on this planet to do. I could feel it in my gut – it's that deep knowing that you might be familiar with. Like your life is going to change whether you want it to or not. I could feel the years slipping away, as they tend to do, and after a series of ignored signs from the universe, it all culminated into the perfect storm a few years ago: all in one day, I left my house, my relationship, my job and even the state I was living in, and returned home, carrying my early twenties midlife crisis with me. What followed was a year of self-discovery – a chance to rebuild myself to become someone I wanted to be, rather than someone I was always told I should be.

Thanks to a number of seriously amazing books and people and some new-found curiosity, I found myself becoming aware of the importance of self-inquiry and of finding something that you love and feel you can share with the world. This led me to my obsession with natural beauty and wellness and encouraged me to develop my own natural beauty business. While I was figuring things out, spending time in nature and developing rituals of self-care were vital for my healing. I found myself wondering how it was possible that nobody had told me just how critical these rituals and a connection to nature are for us humans.

Since this realisation, I have started two companies to provide women with products that help them feel their healthiest, while also enhancing their natural beauty. I'm a total natural beauty and wellness nerd – I'm not ashamed to say it. I'll spend hours researching the most effective ingredients, and I'm doing my best to steer women away from using potentially toxic ingredients found in conventional (non-natural) beauty products. Along with my university degree in media and communications (which, let's be honest, I will probably never use), I have gone a bit left of centre and studied natural and alternative therapies like reiki (if you haven't tried this, you must!), aromatherapy, nutrition and flower essence therapy.

I have seen beauty from all angles and I can tell you, after working with the most beautiful women in the world, that beauty is really about self-love and rituals with a mind–body approach that incorporate how you feel, as well as how healthy and attractive you look. I believe it's time to align our beauty routines with the other wellness practices we follow. Eating healthily and going to the gym is not always a prescription for feeling beautiful, I'm afraid!

Natural beauty is about much more than just using toxin-free products. The roots of herbal healing practices run deep. Just the other week I bathed in a tea tree lake in northern New South Wales. This practice is thought to have been discovered by Indigenous Australians who noticed that bathing in tea tree water could heal wounds. I love the sacred origins of natural rituals and remedies. Modern medicine is lifesaving, but I don't think we should ever forget our connection with nature and the beautifying and healing that nature can provide.

My memories of beauty and wellness go from beautifully emotional to a disastrous mess. From my mum applying lipstick on her way to work, singing 'I say a little prayer for you', to that time I thought it would be a *wonderful* idea to apply an irritant essential oil right under my eyes. Oh, and who could forget the (DIY) coffee enemas! On the other hand, there's my beloved Japanese electro acupuncture (I swear by this!) and the homemade easy-fix beauty treatments you'll be hearing more about soon.

While it all feels a bit surreal that I'm sitting here writing a book for you about beauty and wellness, I don't feel like an impostor. In the pages that lay ahead of you, eagerly waiting to be turned, you'll find some of my personal top beauty tricks, from supermodel secrets to ancient sacred therapies. Everything I share with you is self-taught and from personal experience. I have tried and tested more weird therapies than I can count, and if there are more wellness-related things to do or therapies to try – fun! I'm in. Having said that, there will never be a time where I solemnly swear to forgo eating sugar or drinking wine – I don't think being an extremist at anything is a good idea. But DIY facials? I swear by them. Abhyanga? It's one of my favourite practices (you'll know what this is soon).

I am proud to say I practice what I preach in terms of wellness. It's not about overhauling your lifestyle; it's about small changes that make a big difference in how you look and feel. I hope that with this book you'll not only improve your health and beauty, but develop a relationship with yourself and nature.

My routine

It would hardly be fair to give you all this information without revealing what I really do. Well, let me start by saying my love for lotions and potions knows no limit, so if this sounds overwhelming, then remember: I like to be my own guinea pig. My daily, weekly and monthly routines change every now and then depending on what I need or feel like playing around with. I live by the 80/20 rule: I choose healthy and natural ingredients and products 80 per cent of the time.

In the morning, the first thing I do is clean my tongue with my copper tongue scraper. It's an Ayurvedic health technique. Do this once and you'll be hooked – you won't be able to start your day knowing how much toxin-filled gunk builds up on your tongue overnight. Scraping your tongue helps stimulate gastric and digestive enzymes for the day ahead and gets rid of that nasty morning breath. After this, it's time for oil pulling. I pop a spoonful of coconut oil into my mouth and swish it around for a few minutes before rinsing. Oil pulling is thought to reduce bad breath and the bacteria that cause it, and it has even been reported to help whiten your teeth.

Then it's tea time: my favourite ritual. Usually, it's a hot tea that has digestive benefits. And after tea? My smoothie. My friends affectionately refer to my morning smoothies as 'pond smoothies' because, well, they aren't pretty and often have a lovely tinge of green (thanks, chlorella powder!). My smoothie can contain anywhere between four and ten ingredients. Today, half of my smoothie ended up spilled down my stairs. Nonetheless, it included both pre- and probiotics (following the results from a gut microbiome test), ashwagandha (an Ayurvedic wonder herb for stress), a red vegetable health powder,

vegan hemp protein, vitamin C powder and a bunch of frozen berries. It tastes better than it sounds, I swear.

After my smoothie, it's time for my skincare. I either rinse my face or shower. If I've been exercising in the morning, I apply a magnesium-infused moisturiser after my shower; otherwise I just use rosehip oil or a body oil with detoxing essential oils or vitamin C. I also use a vitamin C serum on my face, neck and décolletage, and let it sink in as I do my hair. Then it's a thick moisturiser over the top of the vitamin C on my face, followed by a SPF lotion, usually in the form of a BB cream. If I am wearing make-up, it's natural (aside from my mascara – I just can't find a great natural one). For my perfume, it's essential oils. Rose geranium is my go-to this month.

At night, I usually remove make-up with an oil. You'll find it binds well to make-up and removes it all like magic. Sometimes I will use a natural micellar water too. I do sometimes wash my face with a natural cleanser, but probably only every second night. I usually apply niacinamide (vitamin B3) serum and a nourishing oil overnight, but I also use an acid (mostly lactic) twice a week or a gentle retinol oil once a week. I make sure everything goes on my décolletage and the back of my hands too. My body doesn't usually need more moisturiser at night, because I normally use an oil-rich exfoliating scrub in the shower.

In terms of my daily supplements, they vary. I find milk thistle removes dark circles from under my eyes and cod liver oil stops my skin from being dry. I also take resveratrol and nicotinamide riboside (NR) for their cell renewing benefits and prevention of premature ageing. If I have a bigger or richer meal than usual, I'll take digestive enzymes.

If I feel bloated, I take oregano oil capsules. They work really well, as do peppermint oil capsules. I love drinking water – it's weird, I know, but I am never without my 1 litre (34 fl oz) bottle, which I refill once or twice a day. I usually drink about four cups of herbal tea per day too. Some have medicinal benefits, some just taste great.

Finally, I would probably lose my mind if I sat inside all day, so I go outside and/or work out every day. My workouts change all the time, from yoga to high-intensity exercise. Vedic meditation is also part of my wellness habit (you'll hear more about this later). Like I said – wellness is beauty, beauty is wellness. I believe in taking a mind–body approach. And if you want to have a wine and some cake, feel free to do that too.

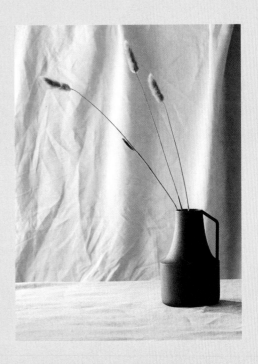

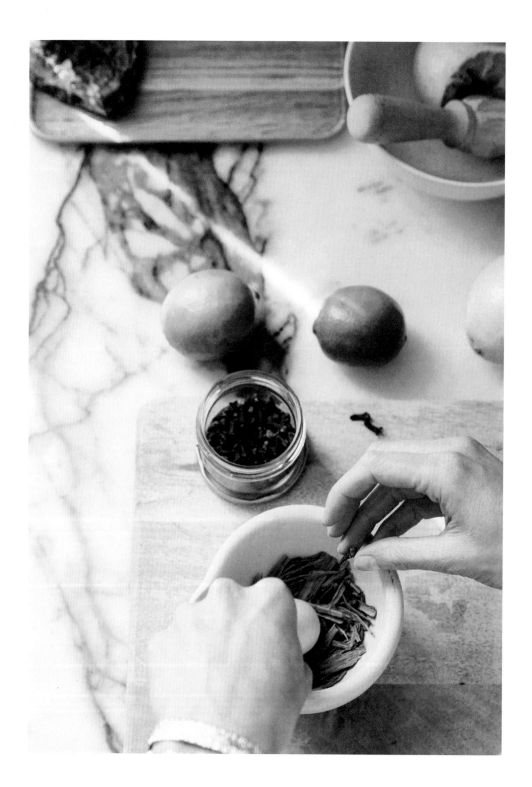

My recipes

For this book, I only wanted to include the most effective yet simplest recipes. In my experience, the more complicated recipes are, the less I make them. Generally, the recipes I've chosen call for a few ingredients only and are easy to make, so you don't need to put too much time and effort aside. The recipes can also be tailored to your personal preference. Want a more or less oily body scrub? Go for it! A lip balm that makes your lips redder? No worries! The ingredients are simple enough that you can tinker around and play with what suits you.

It's worth noting that most recipes made with natural ingredients can last up to three days, excluding the scrubs, which can keep for up to three months. Always store your concoctions in an airtight container and in the fridge if possible.

Toxic ingredients

Why do conventional skincare products and cosmetics use toxic ingredients? They're cheap, easy to work with and readily available. Many of these ingredients are relatively new to market, so they have never been tested for their safety – we are the guinea pigs.

When parabens show up in malignant cancer tissue and the ingredients in make-up and skincare products are also used in things like car-washing detergent, why would you want to use them on yourself? It's not like you're exposed to just one chemical either. It's thought that women expose themselves to an average of 168 chemicals per day from their cosmetics alone.

Think about how many products you use on your face, hair and body, as well as your cleaning products, the artificial preservatives and colours in your food, and the general environmental pollution. As much as autoimmune responses like rashes are annoying and worrying, it's the gradual build-up that does the real damage.

Nature has a solution for almost anything you need, so why use toxic or potentially unsafe conventional ingredients when nature can offer the same benefits without the risk?

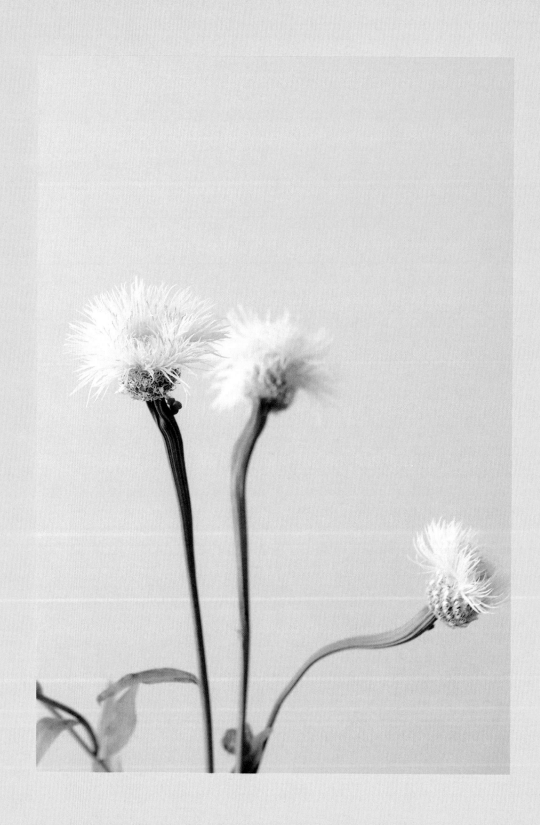

01

Face

The skin on your face goes through a lot. Weather, emotion, hormones – it wears it all.

I don't believe there is any need for a thirteen-step skin routine. Cleanse and moisturise every day. Apply a face mask once or twice per week. Exfoliate. Wear sunscreen. And steer clear of toxic ingredients!

On that note, oils are key for healthy skin too, not just for dry skin. Oils differ from conventional creams, which are full of binders that feel as if they're working, but really are just sitting on top of the skin. Oils have been used in skincare and beauty rituals for centuries, so we know their effectiveness. I use them every day in a million ways, as you'll see.

Top 4 beauty myths

1. 'Hypo-allergenic' means 'safe for everyone'.

2. Collagen can be absorbed topically through skincare.

3. You should aim for squeaky-clean skin.

4. My face cream was $250 so it must be good.

Skin types

To me, the idea of having a single skin type is a controversial concept. There's no perfect type to aim for; it's about seeking balance for our skin. We aren't generally born with just one skin type; our skin can change throughout our lives due to a variety of factors, like our environment, our age and our hormones. That's why it's good to know about each skin type, and not just rely on how it feels today.

I'll cover how to care for dry, oily, sensitive and mature skin. You'll see me mentioning specific ingredients – to include in your diet and to use topically – that are good for each skin type. Along with offering my 100 per cent natural DIY recipes, I'll discuss ingredients that you might be less familiar with, such as the alpha-hydroxy and beta-hydroxy acids we use as chemical exfoliants (page 48).

Tips & Tricks: Your skin might feel dry as you arrive home after a big night out, because your oil production halves at 2 am! That's why using a face oil before bed is a great idea.

Ayurveda

Ayurveda is the ancient wisdom–filled Hindu practice of medicine, and it's believed to be the oldest in the world. In Ayurveda, perfect skin is luminous like the full moon and referred to as prabha. Dull or pale skin is called chaya. Great skin isn't the result of an expensive moisturiser; it's the culmination of the benefits you get from a variety of natural products and treatments, as well as inner contentment and happiness – beauty does show from the inside out.

If you feel like you've tried everything to heal your skin, no matter what the condition, you might want to consider going to an Ayurvedic doctor. They will look at your whole body and mind and give you a prescription of herbs, teas and treatments that will not only benefit your skin, but also your overall health.

Ayurvedic treatments are such a treat. I'll never forget the first time I walked into an Ayurvedic clinic: the walls were adorned with medicinal herb–infused body oils, pretty much my idea of heaven. It was then that I tried my first Ayurvedic skin oil, prescribed to me by quite possibly the healthiest-looking doctor in the world.

Herb and flower facial steam treatment

For: A spa experience for clearer, cleaner skin. The steam opens pores and draws out impurities. The herbs and flowers are bursting with medicinal qualities and skin-purifying and softening effects.

1 tablespoon lavender flowers
1 tablespoon rose petals
1 tablespoon dried chamomile
5–10 fresh mint leaves
1 sprig fresh rosemary

Option: For oily skin, try a combination of 1 tablespoon each of basil, lemon balm, witch hazel and sage.

I've always loved steam rooms, but I have an aversion to using them unless they are spotless, and public steam rooms seem to always be just … not up to scratch. The exception was an experience I'll never forget when I was travelling through Mexico and found a heavenly day spa in Tulum. Placed in the centre of the steam room was a massive collection of herbs. They smelled incredible. Since then, I've been obsessed with combining herbs with steam.

One of the best things about facial steam recipes is that they allow you to create your own sacred spa space at home, giving you a few special minutes of total relaxation. For this recipe, you can use fresh or dried flowers.

To make: Fill a large, wide bowl with boiling water.

Add the flowers and herbs. If you are using fresh flowers, you can reserve some to add later so they look fresh, but this is purely for aesthetic purposes.

Let the flowers and herbs steep for 5 minutes.

To use: Place your face at least 30 cm (12 in) over the bowl with a towel over your head and shoulders to stop steam escaping. Breathe deeply and enjoy for 10 minutes.

Use once or twice per week.

Almond foaming cleanser

For: Skin that wants a fresh clean.

¼ cup castile soap
¾ cup water
1 tablespoon almond oil
3 drops essential oil of your choice

Sometimes milky cleanser just doesn't cut it. This recipe will satisfy your craving for a foaming cleanser. It contains almond oil so it nourishes and feeds your skin, while the castile soap cleans and prevents the almond oil from making your skin oily.

To make: Add all the ingredients to an empty foam dispenser bottle. Shake to combine.

To use: Use in the shower as a face and body wash.

Use daily or nightly – whenever you shower!

Dry skin

First up, let it be known – dry skin and dehydrated skin are different. Dry skin is a skin condition where skin feels and looks visibly dry. You can't miss it. Your skin will be lacking in oils and fats, so supplements like fish oils and a diet rich in healthy fats will help. You might feel like your skin is so dry that it feels tight, or perhaps it's even a little itchy for no apparent reason.

Dehydrated skin is what you'll see when you look in the mirror the morning after a night out. Fine lines are more pronounced and easily fixed by rehydrating and keeping hydrated throughout the day. Steer clear of showers that are too hot and excessive air conditioning. You will also notice that your skin will be more dehydrated on aeroplanes – hellish places for your skin.

Your skin can be dry for a number of reasons. These include allergens, extreme weather conditions, rosacea, vitamin deficiencies or even the cleaning products you use. The good news is that it can be brought back into balance, and it may be even easier than you think. With small changes to your diet and the products you use, you'll be surprised at how quickly your dry skin can return to its healthy state.

There's no arguing about what my skin is like – it's dry. I remember not too long ago: if I forgot to apply my oils or moisturiser, my skin would be so tight it would feel as if I was wearing a clay face mask. And it's not just my face; my body needs just as much attention when it comes to moisturiser. (I often put oil on my body before bed and I'm constantly washing my stained sheets as a result.) I know my dry skin is partly genetic (my dad has dry skin too), but I've also found ways to beat it. And it's not all topical solutions; there are supplements that can help with all skin conditions and changes you can make to your diet, along with using lovely natural lotions and potions.

DRY SKIN NUTRITION

It's not rocket science when we eat to help dry skin. As you might expect, foods that are rich in oils are at the top of your shopping list. Seafood, olive oil, avocados – the more the merrier. Consuming more omega-3 fatty acids is one thing you can do to keep the skin hydrated. These polyunsaturated fatty acids protect the skin from UV exposure, help repair already damaged skin, and keep cell membranes healthy and hydrated. This keeps toxins out and your skin looking supple and soft.

Salmon is your dry skin seafood go-to, because it contains lots of omega-3 fatty acids. I am picky with my salmon; I want to know where it came from, if it was farmed or wild and if it was caught using sustainable fishing methods. Aim for salmon that has been sustainably caught.

There are also plenty of omega-3 rich foods that are vegetarian. However, because most vegetarian sources contain only the alpha-linolenic type of omega-3 fatty acid, consuming a combination of vegetarian and non-vegetarian sources is recommended.

Aside from seaweed – nori, kelp and wakame, to name a few – which has all three types of omega-3 fatty acids, you'll be looking for nuts and seeds such as chia seeds, which are super high in skin-loving omega 3. Hemp seeds are another option and work as a great addition to your breakfast. I add them to smoothies and on top of yoghurt. They have a pretty green flavour, so don't add too much! Nuts have the added benefit of vitamin C; however, they can be hard to digest, so try to buy activated nuts, which are a bit easier to digest. Avocado has omega-9 fatty acids and vitamin A, which has anti-inflammatory properties. The fatty acids help to moisten the skin and reduce inflammation, which often comes hand in hand with dry skin. Avocados also contain sterolin, which can help reduce age spots.

WHAT TO USE TOPICALLY

Your dry skin will love oils. Most plant oils will help, but rosehip and avocado would be particularly beneficial. Avocado oil has been used since Aztec times as a super skin moisturiser that doesn't clog pores. You can use non-comedogenic oils like these both at night and during the day. I even like to mix my moisturisers or serums with oils for an extra nourishing boost. For severely dry skin or for skin that's been whipped by some harsh winter weather, you can make a simple yet effective ointment by experimenting with some plant-based glycerine or castor wax.

Essential oils can be used on dry skin, but make sure you dilute them in a plant oil first, especially if your skin is a little sensitive. The best essential oils for dry skin are patchouli and lavender; dilute them at a ratio of about 1:10 with a plant oil, such as sweet almond or jojoba. Both essential oils have anti-inflammatory properties: patchouli can stimulate the growth of new skin, while lavender can be used to treat minor burns and helps balance the skin's moisture levels. When it comes to face wash, avoid surfactants – soaps, detergents, pretty much anything that foams – these further break up your skin's natural oils. Try micellar water to remove make-up and a cream-based cleanser.

Vitamin C products (page 54) can be drying on skin, so use them sparingly if you choose to at all. Vitamin C is thought to be activated by sunlight, and because it helps protect your skin from UV light and pollution, it's best used in the morning.

If you choose to exfoliate, use a gentle lactic acid (which is effective for removing the dead top layer of your skin) and don't go overboard. You can build up to using chemical exfoliants more regularly. Physical exfoliation is fine, especially with gentle scrubs that contain moisturising ingredients and oils. (There's more information on exfoliation on pages 46–48.)

Niacinamide is an active ingredient that will be soothing on your skin whilst helping to strengthen the skin's barrier. You can mix it with a very gentle retinol product, such as retinyl palmitate, and use it at night. (There's more on these ingredients on pages 53–54.)

Hyaluronic acid is reputed to be wonderful for dry skin, although I personally didn't notice a great difference when I used it. Worth a try though!

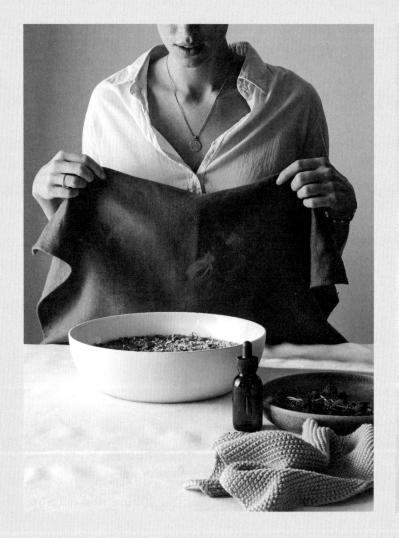
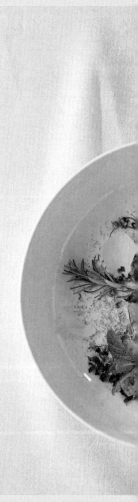

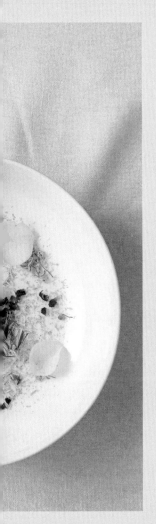

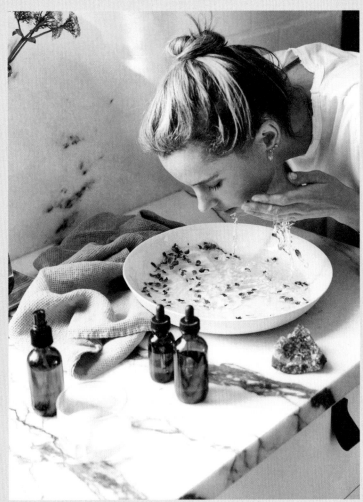

You'll know by now the importance of consuming enough fatty acids for your skin. From here, it's all about moisturising day and night, using anti-inflammatory niacinamide (page 54), and applying a face mask once or twice per week.

- **Daytime:** Your best option is an oil-based serum. You can also use a rich moisturiser or a simple plant oil with a lighter moisturiser.

- **Daytime actives:** Use a vitamin C product (page 54) and/or hyaluronic acid. Because vitamin C can be drying, use it sparingly.

- **Night-time:** Try an oil-based serum such as jojoba or rosehip with a couple of drops of essential oils.

- **Night-time actives:** Apply a niacinamide cream (you can mix it with your oil for extra nourishment). Avoid using retinol if you have very dry skin. Bakuchiol is an effective, non-drying retinol alternative for dry or sensitive skin. (There's more on these ingredients on pages 53–54.)

- **Weekly or more often:** Apply a hydrating face mask, like the Honey and rosewater mask (page 35), and use an oil-rich scrub, like the Brown sugar vanilla dessert scrub (page 76) on your body.

- **Twice a week:** Use a chemical exfoliant (page 48).

Don't forget to up your omegas! Taking cod liver oil (as gross as it sounds) as a supplement really is the best thing I have done for my dry skin. If you prefer, vegan alternatives, such as chia seed or flaxseed oil, are also available.

Tips & Tricks: Instead of using a toner to remove make-up, use an oil. Lots of skin and make-up products are oil based, and the best thing for cleansing oil off your face is another oil! Castor oil is a heavy oil that is great at removing make-up when mixed with a more viscous oil like avocado. Just combine 2 parts avocado oil and 1 part castor oil. Pop it onto a cotton pad and wipe over your face to remove make-up.

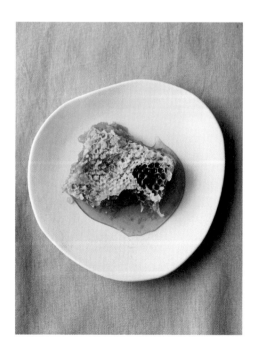

Oily and acne-prone skin

We've all been there. The cliché of waking up with a pimple on the day of a party. Often a stubborn pimple, accompanied by many others. We've also tried all the creams and potions, but to no avail. Whether it's on your face or your butt, there are lots of natural tricks that are effective in both preventing and stopping the pimples in their tracks.

Ever wondered how your skin gets so clear when you take a beach holiday? Maybe it's the decrease in stress levels, maybe it's the antibacterial properties of the sun ... but it's probably the salt water working its magic and restoring your skin. It's true – salt is a natural pimple-busting beauty hack. It naturally removes excess oil and has antibacterial powers. You can make a little saltwater potion for the rest of the year when you're not on a beach holiday to help clear your skin: combine 1 teaspoon of sea salt with a couple of teaspoons of hot water. Don't worry if the salt doesn't fully dissolve – just dab the solution on the problem area at bedtime and you'll notice a big difference. As for the best active ingredients to get rid of pimples, choose salicylic or glycolic acid (page 48) as a spot treatment, but use them sparingly.

....

Tips & Tricks: Adding a couple of drops of tea tree oil to the salty water will help clear super stubborn spots and will also increase the antibacterial properties of the mixture.

Acne and pimples can be triggered by a range of things: poor digestion, candida overgrowth, vitamin or mineral deficiencies, hormonal imbalance and our skincare products and make-up. Our skin is trying to fit into a world where we are exposed to toxins, processed foods, pharmaceutical drugs, concentrated hormones in our food and an overabundance of sugar. Our skin can be like a volcano; when we fill our bodies to their toxin-holding capacity, our skin (our body's largest organ) lets us know. I don't believe that the innate intelligence of our bodies would give us symptoms for no reason at all. That's why I don't agree with only masking the symptoms of the problem, like slapping some concealer on the pimples that you've had for months (although as a temporary solution, I get it). You can work on getting rid of the symptoms while figuring out what's happening internally by going on your own detective adventure – either by yourself or with a naturopath, doctor or dermatologist.

OILY AND ACNE-PRONE SKIN NUTRITION

We should try to remember that if acne is caused by a hormonal imbalance, for example, then the pimples will continue to rear their heads until the real cause is addressed. I had a strange rash on the back of my shoulders a few years ago that looked like it was some kind of fungal infection: the skin was losing its pigmentation in small areas. I removed all inflammatory foods from my diet, stopped eating fructose, and within three days the rash was gone, never to be seen again. This is what worked for me, but what works for you might take some time to figure out.

Diet can have a dramatic impact on your skin, and there is a link between dairy intake and acne. Low glycaemic index–diets have been shown to help reduce acne, so you might want to give that a go. I find a diet that isn't too high in carbohydrates, or too heavy in red meats, keeps me energetic and functioning to the best of my ability.

Hydration's just as important when you have oily skin and pimples. Many of us try to avoid anything containing oil when we have oily skin or even just a few pimples; we all think that anything heavy blocks our pores. But if you do suffer from acne, you might actually want to try oils in your skincare regime.

Not all oils are comedogenic, or pore clogging. Applying oils to your face can balance your oil production and help clear your skin. Sometimes when we strip our skin of oils, we only end up making our skin produce excessive amounts of oil, leaving us more prone to acne. You might also find after stripping the oils from your skin that the top layer is dry and flaky while the skin below remains oily.

Try jojoba oil – it is known for its non-comedogenic properties. Use jojoba oil at night or to remove make-up. Grapeseed is another plant oil you might want to make use of, and you can swap this in for any recipes containing coconut oil (which is comedogenic). Last but not least, tamanu oil has antibacterial properties, so this is a well-suited option too.

Traditional anti-ageing ingredients retinol and other retinoids (page 53) can also help reduce acne and increase cell turnover – just be sure to use them only at night and apply a sunscreen during the day as they increase the skin's sensitivity to the sun.

There are plenty of beauty treatments that you can do at home. Don't feel like you can't apply a face mask just because you have acne. If you really are averse to using oil (though you shouldn't be), try a clay mask. There are many different types of clays that love oily skin, and they all have an anti-inflammatory effect and can help draw out impurities from pimple-prone skin. Bentonite clay is thought of as the best for oily skin. It's rich in silica and effectively pulls toxins from the skin. When you buy raw, dry bentonite clay powder, it shouldn't have any other ingredients. You'll need to mix it with a liquid to make a paste. Other natural beauty ingredients such as soothing aloe vera and detoxifying charcoal are also ideal for oily or pimple-prone skin.

In terms of essential oils for oily or acne-prone skin, you'll be using tea tree a lot. It's one of the most versatile essential oils out there, and a very effective spot treatment for pimples. If your skin can tolerate it, toners with witch hazel or tea tree will be great for you. Be careful with these though, as they can make any open wounds sting. Make your own toner using 3 tablespoons of witch hazel, 2 tablespoons of water and 4 drops of tea tree oil, and mist your face (with your eyes closed) or body when you wake up or after a shower.

Floral waters are pre-blended solutions of essential oils and water. If you're looking for a more beneficial floral water, opt for a hydrosol, which is the liquid collected from flowers during the steam distillation process that turns them into essential oils. If you're a fan of lavender, it's a great floral water or hydrosol for oily skin to use as a mist or in a body or face oil. You can make a little pillow spray with it too. Lavender oil is known for its scar-healing benefits and works well with oily skin, making it perfect for any acne scars.

For exfoliants, apple-cider vinegar contains a blend of gentle acids, such as acetic and lactic, which work together for a natural exfoliating effect. Apple-cider vinegar is also known to balance pH (that's why some people drink it in the morning) and provide antibacterial effects. Test it out by using only a little first! I once got a rash all over my face from applying too much of this to my dry skin. Salicylic acid is another chemical exfoliant that you might find works better for your skin and is great for reducing pimples. (Read more on chemical exfoliants on page 48.) Oily skin usually isn't as sensitive as other skin types, so you have more freedom with choosing the ingredients you use.

Vitamin C products (page 54) can work for all skin types to reduce signs of premature ageing. After a face mask, you may want to also try blue light therapy. The blue light is thought to kill the bacteria causing breakouts. Lots of salons offer this treatment at the end of facials as an add-on, but you can also buy a device to use at home.

THE OILY AND ACNE-PRONE SKIN ROUTINE

Chances are you'll experience oily skin at some stage in your life. I find I can get oily skin on my upper back, a particularly hard spot to treat without extra long, bendy arms. It's about keeping your skin clean to help reduce and prevent acne, without over-stripping it of its oils.

- **Daytime:** Don't be scared of moisturisers; a light moisturiser for day use is totally safe for your pimple-prone skin. Apply this after a vitamin C serum or oil (page 54). Use a foaming natural cleanser, such as the Almond foaming cleanser (page 17), or cleanse with a micellar water and an oil.

- **Daytime actives:** Vitamin K is your friend; pimples often come hand in hand with inflammation and redness, which vitamin K can help with. Vitamin C is a great all-rounder, and can have a gentle drying effect and reduce acne scars.

- **Night-time:** A small amount of tamanu oil can be used on your skin, along with a serum containing vitamin K.

- **Night-time actives:** Retinol or retinoid-based products (page 53) can work well for pimple-prone skin, as they not only work on softening pigmentation and wrinkles, but also reduce acne. Avoid using these products with your chemical exfoliants (page 48).

- **Weekly or more often:** Apply a face mask (clay ones are great – try the Moroccan-inspired mud mask on page 28) and use the scrubs on page 77 on your body.

- **Twice a week:** Use an exfoliant on your face (pages 46–48) to help reduce acne scarring. Salicylic acid can be used up to five times a week.

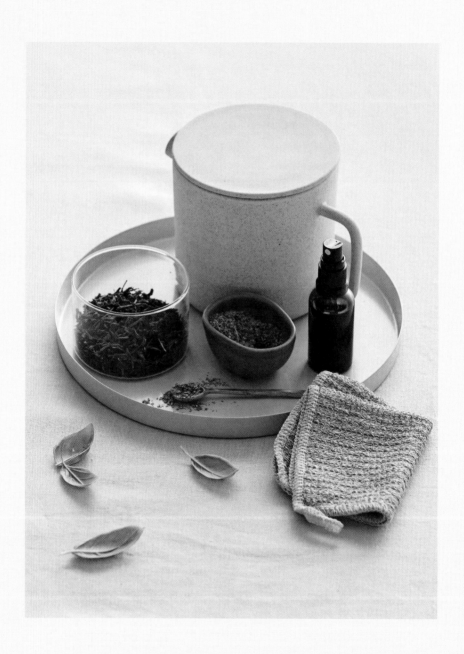

Basil, tea tree and green tea anti–acne toner

For: Clarifying and toning pimple-prone skin.

This antioxidant-rich toner is full of antibacterial goodness and pimple-fighting ingredients. It might feel odd using basil in the bathroom when it's usually reserved for the kitchen, but it has great health properties for acne-prone skin. You'll also hear me going on about tea tree over and over. It's the one ingredient that's always in my house; I use it for cleaning and for pimples and rashes. The smell reminds me so much of my home country and holidays spent in nature.

1½ cups water
3 tablespoons dried basil leaves
2 green tea bags
4 drops tea tree oil

To make: Bring the water to a boil in a saucepan. Add the basil and green tea bags and let them infuse into the water for 1 hour.

Remove the tea bags, strain out the basil leaves and transfer the infused water to a mist spray bottle.

Add the tea tree oil and shake to combine.

To use: Use on a cotton pad as a toner at night. You can also mist on your face upon waking – just have your eyes closed.

Use daily.

Moroccan–inspired mud mask

For: Pimple-prone skin.

½ cup rhassoul mud powder
⅓ cup rose hydrosol or
   rosewater
2 drops rose essential oil

Option: If you have dry skin, you might want to swap the rhassoul mud for pink clay.

You can substitute rose essential oil with rosewood oil or buy a diluted version; these are more affordable – just remember to double the quantity.

Clay is super clarifying and great for oily or acne-prone skin. It draws out impurities and has a detoxing effect. You can use any type of cosmetic mud, but this one uses silky rhassoul mud.

To make: Pour the mud powder into a bowl and give it a quick stir to make sure it doesn't have any clumps.

Start adding the rose hydrosol gradually while stirring the mixture.

Once all the rose hydrosol is thoroughly mixed in, add the rose essential oil.

To use: Apply the mask to clean dry skin on your face and neck. Leave on for 20 minutes, then rinse thoroughly. Moisturise with a face oil afterwards. This mixture will likely give you a couple of uses, so store the remainder in an airtight container for up to 3 days.

Apply once or twice a week.

Sensitive skin

Sensitive skin and dry skin can often be found together, and they both require a delicate touch and some extra TLC. Over-scrubbing, over-cleansing and even environmental pollution can contribute to your sensitive skin, so the thing you need to remember more than anything is to go easy.

....

Tips & Tricks: A humidifier in your bedroom can do wonders for dry or sensitive skin in winter. You can add some essential oils and sleep with it on at night.

SENSITIVE SKIN NUTRITION

Is your skin dry too? Your skin acts as a barrier, but dry, cracked skin allows irritants to easily penetrate, so it's important to look after it with nourishing oils and moisturisers, and consume lots of healthy fats in your diet. Cutting out dairy, processed foods and refined sugar as much as possible can be as important as what you put on your face. Your skin will thank you. You might also want to eat more acerola cherries. They are one of the richest sources of vitamin C and rutin, a bioflavonoid good for broken capillaries and rosacea, conditions us sensitive skin bunnies often suffer form. Asparagus is another good source of rutin.

Turmeric is great for skin due to its incredible anti-inflammatory properties. It's one of the things I used to add to my DIY rescue face mask, along with honey, to get rid of some dermatitis I had a few years ago around my mouth and nose. Eating or drinking dried or fresh turmeric helps fight inflammation in the body, keeping skin looking fresher and younger, while also helping relieve more serious inflammatory skin problems, such as eczema and rosacea. Inflammation in the body is rough on skin: it speeds up ageing and leads to wrinkles in the long term, and it makes skin look puffy and tired in the short term. You can mix turmeric and rice powder together for a gentle exfoliating paste. According to the *Dongui Bogam*, a book about traditional Korean medicine that was published in 1613, mixing ground mung beans, adzuki beans and soybeans into a powder called jodu makes an excellent facial cleanser. Combine a teaspoon of each powder along with half a teaspoon of turmeric, for a gentle and anti-inflammatory cleanser: massage the mixture on your face while in the shower and your skin will be lovely and soft afterwards.

WHAT TO USE TOPICALLY

In terms of botanicals or floral waters for sensitive skin, calendula and cucumber are extra soothing and can be mixed with rose and lavender essential oils, both of which are generally tolerated in small doses by sensitive skin. German chamomile is a beautiful, safe essential oil for sensitive skin. If you have very sensitive skin, you should avoid essential oils altogether and opt for rose hydrosol, which is like a high-grade rosewater. I use rose hydrosol mist on my face when I wake up. Nothing like the smell of fresh roses to put you in the right mood to start your day!

For ultra sensitive skin, avoid alpha-hydroxy acids (page 48) and retinoids (page 53). You can use a plant-based retinol alternative called bakuchiol, which doesn't come with the irritating effects of retinol. It's a new ingredient on the scene, but it is effective. You'll also want to avoid harsh cleansers in the shower, which disturb the skin's microbiome. You don't need to wash your face in the morning; it will be an unnecessary disruption for your skin.

Sensitive skin can often benefit from healthy, fatty plant oils, especially when used in place of a conventional moisturiser. Apply the oil on damp skin, when it's more porous. When choosing plant oils to use, you're best to avoid nut oils and stick to oils like argan and olive oil. However, you may find that you don't have a problem with most plant oils, so it's really your choice. Camellia oil is hypo-allergenic and reputed to have been used for centuries in Japan as a beauty secret. It comes from the *Camellia oleifera* plant, also known as the 'rose of winter'. Not only can you use it directly on your skin and hair, but it's also great in baths. Make sure your bath isn't too hot though, as hot water can irritate your skin.

Anything that is formulated to help calm redness and irritation will help comfort your sensitive skin. Zinc oxide, a mineral sunscreen, is doubly beneficial as it protects you from the sun and is soothing. I also find calendula-based natural nappy rash creams great for irritated skin.

SENSITIVE SKIN IRRITANTS

We all get sensitive skin at some point. Depending on how sensitive your skin can be, you might even need to avoid some natural ingredients, such as essential oils, altogether. Some essential oils can bring on irritation more than others: lemon and the citrus family of oils smell amazing, but they can also be quite irritating. As can cinnamon and black pepper (yes, that's an essential oil!). Lavender and rose, on the other hand, are known to be calming, so you might find that they are much better for your skin. Don't forget to be safe and dilute the essential oils with a plant oil like jojoba before applying them to your skin.

Synthetic fragrance should absolutely be avoided, because these chemical concoctions are a major allergy starter. Ever experienced nausea or a headache when you smelled a perfume or a scented candle? Yup – that's your body telling you to *step away*. Scented candles are not made with essential oils, nor can they be. Instead, settle for some unscented beeswax candles and an essential oil humidifier. (Essential oil burners tend to damage the composition of the essential oils, so avoid them.)

There are all sorts of blood tests and DNA tests you can get nowadays to determine exactly what your body is sensitive to, if anything at all. For example, you might find that you get a stuffy nose when you go to bed because you're allergic to the laundry detergent you use or the down that fills your pillow. Yes – these tests can figure out all the intricacies for you. I've had many done myself, and although they aren't cheap, they are useful.

Inside out

Everything that burdens our system – whether it be exposure to chemicals or emotional turmoil – must be released by our bodies. The skin happens to be one of the ways our body expels these things – and it's sure one way to get our attention. It all makes sense when you think about it. Our faces show how we feel. Fatigue can show up as dark circles under the eyes and dehydration as pronounced wrinkles and skin that doesn't bounce back. We can even see psychological stress and food intolerances from looking at the skin, particularly with the help of a great naturopath or holistic dermatologist. It could be a mild allergic response to a type of food you keep eating or a diet too rich in salt and heavy carbohydrates. If you've ever had too much to drink and woken up with a pimple or a puffy face, you'll know what I'm talking about.

Recently I went on a month-long holiday and hedonistically ate and drank my way through Spain and Italy. I thought I had dodged a bullet – no stomach issues or skin problems ... that is, until I arrived home and brought with me two large pimples that stayed on my forehead for over a month to remind me to go easy on the cocktails and ice cream. I'm not saying you should not indulge sometimes, but there are ways to protect your beauty and prevent your skin from freaking out.

Our skin really does deserve a bit of extra TLC. After all, it's not just protecting our internal tissue from the environment but also stopping us from becoming dehydrated, protecting us from environmental pathogens, regulating our temperature, synthesising vitamin D and storing vitamins, all while excreting toxins through our sweat. In developed countries, we are lucky enough to have an on-demand supply of clean drinking water; staying hydrated is imperative for beautiful skin. I drink from a jug with a filter that removes toxic metals and fluoride from the drinking water. If I'm dehydrated, I notice it almost immediately by looking at my skin.

Yes – you'll need to take special precautions if your skin is feeling (and acting) a little sensitive, but you'll find it doesn't take extra effort. And sensitive skin issues can often be temporary, anyway. There are some ingredients you'll want to be a little wary of, such as alpha-hydroxy acids (page 48), but there are plenty of more gentle alternatives, so don't feel like you're missing out!

- **Daytime:** Avoid hot water in the morning, which can irritate your skin. Opt for lukewarm instead, or simply mist your face with rose hydrosol or mineral-rich water when you wake up. A light, natural moisturiser will be all you need, and a zinc oxide–based sunscreen can also double as a sensitive skin helper, so apply some of that as well.

- **Daytime actives:** If you have really sensitive skin, you'll need to be careful with active ingredients. A vitamin K–rich serum helps reduce skin redness.

- **Night-time:** Focus on using a calming oil like apricot or camellia oil.

- **Night-time actives:** You should be fine using a niacinamide serum or cream, which can help with inflammation and rosacea. It can also help with hyperpigmentation, which is useful, as you won't be able to use retinol products. You can use bakuchiol as an alternative to retinol; it has been shown to slow signs of premature ageing. (There's more on these ingredients on pages 53–54.)

- **Weekly or more often:** Practise a facial steam treatment (page 17) with chamomile or calendula flowers. Apply a face mask with nourishing ingredients (for example, you can try the Honey and rosewater mask on page 35). Avoid conventional products with fragrance and other hidden irritants. Use a scrub (page 74) but on your body only.

- **Twice a week:** If your skin isn't too sensitive, you can try chemical exfoliants (page 48). Use an alpha-hydroxy acid, such as lactic acid at 5-10 per cent, but this should be avoided if you feel your skin isn't strong enough yet. You can start with the Berry enzyme mask (page 51) that'll give you the same benefits without the irritation. Try to avoid beta-hydroxy acids to begin with. When your skin gets more used to acids, you can try betaine salicylate (a gentler beta-hydroxy acid) at 2 per cent or salicylic acid at 0.5 per cent.

....

Tips & Tricks: Rice water (the water strained from boiled rice and then cooled) is thought to have been used by Japanese women for centuries. It contains vitamins such as B1, C and E, as well as minerals, which together can shrink pores. It can be massaged into the skin like a mini facial before being rinsed off. You can even mix it with rice bran powder, which is high in sterols, to encourage cell regeneration.

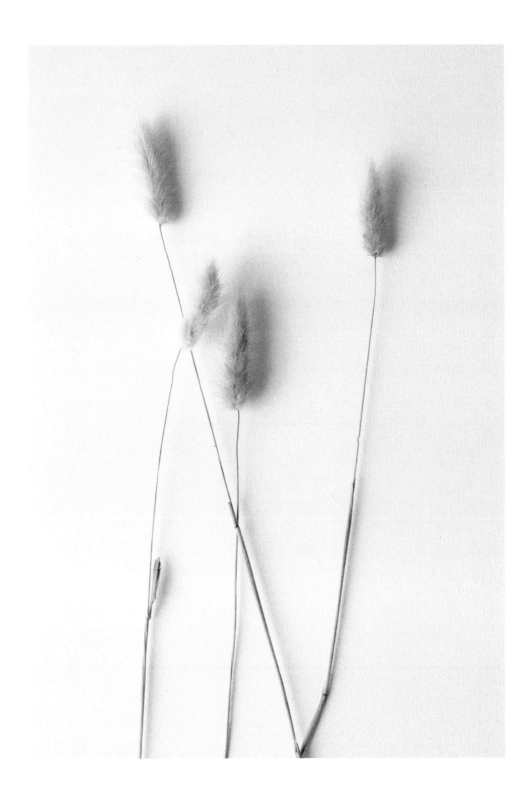

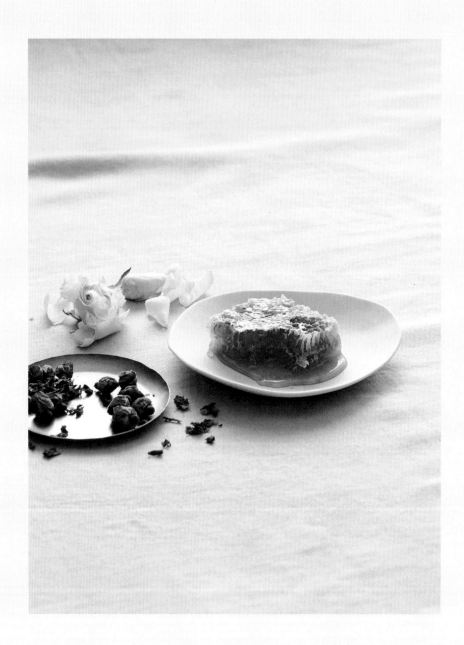

Honey and rosewater mask

For: Sensitive skin.

1 tablespoon honey
  (preferably manuka)
¼ cup rosewater or rose
  hydrosol (hydrosol contains
  more healing elements)

Honey has been used in natural beauty since the days Cleopatra walked the earth. It's thought that she used to luxuriously bathe in honey and milk, with the lactic acid in milk smoothing her royal skin.

I love using a honey face mask while bathing in a coconut milk bath. It feels like total luxury and the honey mask is super calming on your skin. This is one of the most simple and effective DIY face masks I know of. I've also found that honey helps with rashes. I used it daily to help get rid of some perioral dermatitis a few years ago.

Rosewater and rose hydrosol are soothing and hydrating. Keep some in a bottle by your bedside and mist your face when you wake up.

To make: Combine the ingredients in a bowl.

To use: Apply the mask to a clean face and leave on for 20 minutes. The mixture can be quite liquidy, so apply it with a cotton bud or make-up brush if you need. Rinse with warm water and pat dry.

Apply weekly.

Anti-inflammatory turmeric mask

For: Itchy or red skin, particularly pimple-prone skin.

If you haven't heard about the superfood benefits of turmeric, you have surely been living under a rock. This anti-inflammatory wonder herb can go in everything from your smoothie to your face mask.

Turmeric contains curcumin, a potent antioxidant. It has been used in India for centuries in both cooking and medicine, and it's thought to be linked to the country's low rates of bowel cancer. On the skin, turmeric is a natural antiseptic and helps even out skin tone. I've found it very effective for reducing inflammation, especially when it's related to pimples.

½ ripe banana
1 teaspoon turmeric powder
½ teaspoon honey

To make: In a bowl, mash the banana with a fork. Mix in the turmeric powder and honey and stir until combined.

To use: Apply the mask to a clean face and neck and leave on for 15 minutes before washing off.

Use once or twice a week.

Caution! Turmeric stains. Be careful with what you are wearing when you use this mask (or just go nude). If you're using a light-coloured towel, it'll stain that too!

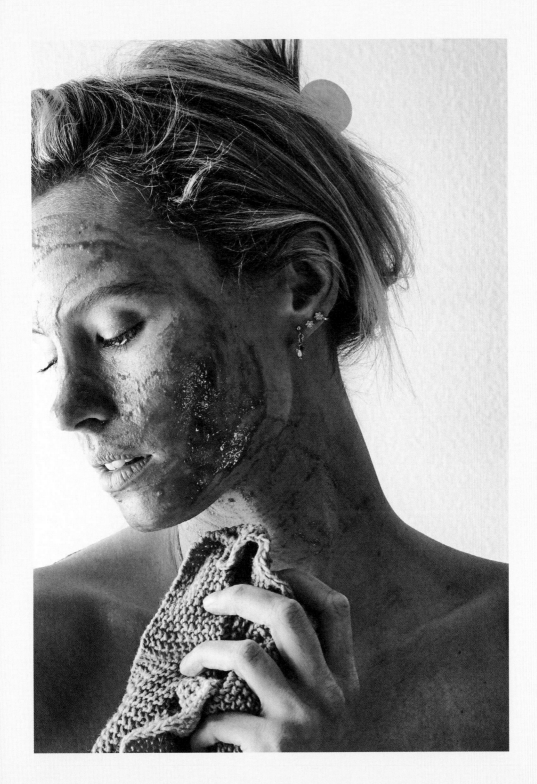

Mature skin

I am not against ageing. I think wrinkles are beautiful and interesting. I have not had, nor do I plan to have, cosmetic procedures (anti-wrinkle injections, fillers etc.), so I won't be able to comment on those. As we age, we can all expect our skin to naturally increase in wrinkles. The ageing process includes slower cell reproduction, deterioration of collagen and elastin, and hormonal changes. But the degree at which our skin ages is somewhat within our control. There is nothing wrong with wrinkles whatsoever, but an inside–out approach to beauty can help prevent ageing quicker and faster than you'd like. In my opinion, the food we eat, what we drink, the supplements we take *and* the products we use on our skin all contribute to ageing factors.

Mature skin needs a boost, from nutrition to moisturisers and exfoliants. Ever noticed how smooth a baby's skin is? This is partly due to their rapid skin cell turnover. The older we get, the slower our skin cell turnover becomes. Ingredients such as alpha-hydroxy acids and salicylic acid (page 48), along with vitamin C (page 54), can all make a serious difference in reducing the signs of ageing. On the other hand, toxic chemicals in conventional skincare products should be avoided as they can stop our skin cells from reproducing as quickly, and thicken the top layer of the epidermis as a result.

MATURE SKIN NUTRITION

Supercharging your diet with antioxidant-rich foods (page 42), helps deactivate cheeky free radicals before they have a chance to harm your healthy skin cells and destroy collagen. Vitamin C-rich foods, blueberries, kale, artichokes and herbal teas of the white and green varieties are all high in antioxidants. Damage caused by free radicals isn't irreversible. Antioxidants, such as lycopene and vitamin C in tomatoes and the rich nutrients found in oils, can reverse sun damage and other factors contributing to prematurely ageing skin. Of course, you'll also want to use a mineral sunscreen to minimise further damage.

WHAT TO USE TOPICALLY

Exfoliating mature skin is going to be more on the chemical side rather than physical; alpha-hydroxy acids and plant enzymes such as papain will be very useful (read more on exfoliation on pages 46–48). Vitamin A and retinoids (page 53) are also crucial to keeping premature ageing at bay.

I learned about a magical combination of essential oils for mature skin from a model in her fifties who looks like she's still in her early thirties. She swore by carrot seed, frankincense and geranium essential oils. This is a pretty potent combination, and while I think there are benefits, I wouldn't suggest putting it on sensitive skin. For other skin types, I would dilute it in a plant oil, such as borage seed and evening primrose oil. These are great for mature skin and can be used all over your face and body. Apricot kernel oil is another favourite – it's high in oleic fatty acids and easily absorbed into skin.

If you don't mind needles, there's even facial acupuncture for cosmetic purposes, although finding a clinic that specialises in this treatment can be difficult. I've tried it, but I can't comment too much on its effectiveness as a couple of months of treatment are generally required and to be honest, well, I just don't have the patience. I can assure you though, it doesn't hurt a bit (unlike the Japanese acupuncture I put myself through, where the needles are gently electrocuted to stimulate muscles – ouchy, but very good for sore muscle relief). It's thought that cosmetic facial acupuncture stimulates the muscles, helping to firm and tighten skin whilst also boosting circulation and collagen production, to keep skin plump and supple. If you're looking for a less invasive treatment, red light therapy is thought to halt the signs of ageing. You can buy at-home devices or go to a salon. In my experience, you're better off going to a salon. I bought an at-home light device and I have used it twice in probably a year. Not one of my wisest investments.

HYPERPIGMENTATION

Ever noticed blotchy darker patches on your skin? You're looking at hyperpigmentation, also known as melasma, which can be caused by several factors, from sun damage and inflammation to the contraceptive pill.

When the dark patches of pigmentation are found on your forehead, cheeks, lips and nose, it's thought that they are most commonly the result of a hormonal imbalance; pigment cells can be triggered by heightened hormone levels. These are common during pregnancy. Fortunately, there are laser treatments available for hormonal pigmentation, as well as niacinamide (page 54). But you needn't worry too much, as most of the time hyperpigmentation disappears once hormone levels normalise.

Hyperpigmentation loves inflamed, oily skin where the melanin distribution is uneven. Facial waxing or going in the sun after a laser treatment can make you more susceptible.

You'll want to make exfoliation your best friend to lessen hyperpigmentation caused by damaged skin, and work with niacinamide, which is great for inflammation. Your best defence against hyperpigmentation

caused by the sun will be applying a broad-spectrum mineral sunscreen and a vitamin C serum (page 54) in the daytime, and having a night-time regimen of treatments with pigmentation-scavenging ingredients, such as licorice, or vitamin A serums (page 53).

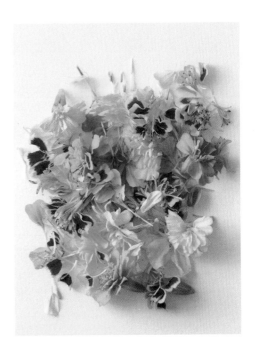

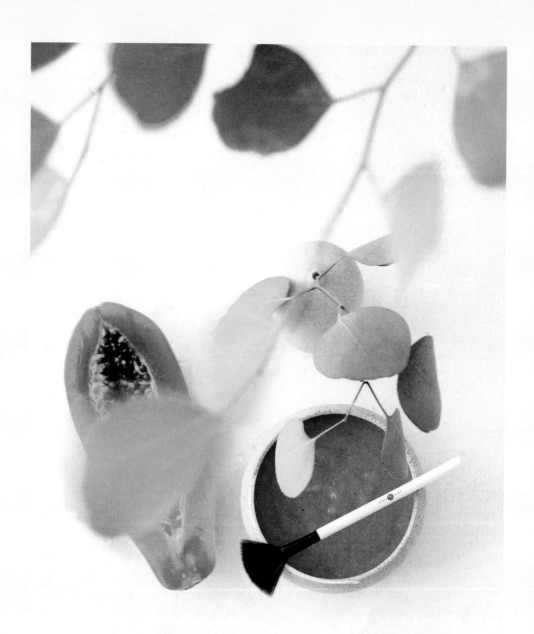

Papaya and pineapple mask

For: Reducing dark spots and pigmentation, as well as helping slough off dead skin.

½ fresh papaya, peeled and seeded
1 cup diced fresh pineapple

Nothing gives me the tropical feels like this mask. It reminds me of mornings in Bali eating half a papaya with lime for breakfast before hopping on a motorbike and going exploring.

Unripe papaya contains natural exfoliating alpha-hydroxy acids and high levels of papain, a dead-skin-dissolving enzyme. (When we eat it, papain helps us digest food.) Pineapple has lots of the enzyme bromelain, which helps remove the outer layers of skin and increase cell turnover.

To make: Blitz the papaya and pineapple together in a blender.

To use: Apply the mixture to a clean face, neck and décolletage. Leave on for 20 minutes. If it tingles a little, that's normal! It's doing what it's meant to do. Rinse with water and moisturise afterwards.

Use once or twice a week.

Resveratrol wine toner

For: Ageing skin.

⅓ cup rosewater or sugar-free aloe vera juice
3 teaspoons good-quality red wine

I couldn't not add wine to one of these recipes. Not only do I love drinking a glass of red wine, but it's also great for your skin. The resveratrol in red wine is the queen of youth-boosting ingredients, an anti-ageing powerhouse that you can buy in supplement form too. Aloe vera is soothing and an antiseptic, giving your skin a good clean with a gentle instant facelift.

To make: Combine the ingredients in a mist spray bottle.

To use: Mist over your face, neck and décolletage, with your eyes closed. Let it soak for 10 minutes before rinsing it off.

Use weekly.

Caution! Don't spritz this if you are wearing white clothes or near your white sheets!

So you know these are good for mature skin, but exactly what do they do and how do you make the most of them? Our hedonistic behaviours increase the number of free radicals in our system that can speed up the ageing process. Drinking alcohol, eating lots of sugar and lying in the sun all contribute to free radicals, as do environmental factors and pollutants. Free radicals begin their damage during the naturally occurring process of oxidation. As oxidation begins, electrons, which like to be in pairs, are moved from one molecule to another. The bonds between electrons can break, thereby changing the state of the molecules. When molecules no longer have their electrons in pairs, they are referred to as free radicals. Antioxidants, such as vitamin C, throw water on the fire of oxidation: they come in and lend electrons to pair with free radicals, stabilising the situation and stopping a chain reaction. Without antioxidants, oxidation occurs without interruption and we age more prematurely.

Not only do these antioxidants work on a surface level to beautify your skin, but they also help shield you against skin cancer. Generally, the more colour the vegetable has, the higher its antioxidant levels, so make friends with beetroot, sweet potato, broccoli and berries. You can also find high levels of antioxidants in white and green tea (careful not to heat the water above 80°C), as well as in herbs and spices, such as turmeric, which can credit its main component, curcumin, for its effectiveness. Cloves (yes, that dried herb you hardly ever use) are the ultimate antioxidants and you can make a tea with them.

Incorporate antioxidants into your skincare by way of at-home skin treatments, not just in your diet. Many of the recipes in this book contain these ingredients.

Quality matters when it comes to the produce you consume and the vitamins you buy. Pesticides can increase oxidation, so organic is best where possible.

10 best sources of antioxidants

1. Cloves
2. Sumac
3. Cinnamon
4. Sorghum bran
5. Oregano
6. Turmeric
7. Acai berry
8. Cacao powder
9. Cumin
10. Maqui berry

A healthy diet rich in vegetables and healthy fats is the best thing you can do to fill your body (and skin) with antioxidants, but you can also get them as supplements. Vitamins A, C and E are the ones that you'll want to pay attention to. You can of course put them straight onto your skin in the form of oils or serums, or you can take them as supplements. If you're like me, you'll do both! There are other supplements that you can take but, honestly, if your diet is healthy with plenty of fresh fruit and (predominantly) vegetables, you shouldn't need to. If you think you're lacking in a specific vitamin, get tested before supplementing, otherwise you may end up literally flushing your investment down the toilet (sometimes an excess of vitamins, like the B vitamins, will be excreted in your urine).

MATURE SKIN ROUTINE

Serums, balms, DIY face masks and other concentrated products will be your best bet in caring for your mature skin. Your skin now needs more than just a moisturiser and a cleanser. Natural products can be formulated to be much more targeted and concentrated than regular skincare products that you might buy in a supermarket or at a chemist. Ingredients like retinol (page 53), coenzyme Q10 and hyaluronic acid will also help to stop your skin from ageing prematurely. Specifically formulated blends of active ingredients, along with beneficial botanical extracts, vitamins and antioxidants, can help encourage healthy cell turnover and a reduction in pigmentation and sun spots.

- **Daytime:** My beautiful mum swears by bursting a vitamin E capsule and smearing that on her skin first thing every morning. Follow this with an oil-rich moisturiser.

- **Daytime actives:** Vitamin C products (page 54) are an essential for helping reduce pigmentation, so it's a must for ageing skin if you're looking to keep pigmentation at bay.

- **Night-time:** Oils are your best friend; they help plump up skin. A nourishing eye product, such as the Coffee and arnica eye balm (page 63), can be used nightly.

- **Night-time actives:** Oils can be mixed with a retinoid-based product (page 53).

- **Weekly or more often:** Treat yourself to a facial steam treatment (page 17) with chamomile or calendula flowers. Apply a face mask rich in natural alpha-hydroxy acids, like the Papaya and pineapple mask (page 41), and use a scrub, like the Skin-softening and anti-inflammatory matcha

and avocado oil scrub (page 75), on your body. Nourishing face masks full of plumping ingredients, such as honey (you can try my Honey and rosewater mask on page 35), and naturally exfoliating ingredients, such as berries (use the Berry enzyme mask on page 51), are crucial.

- **Twice a week:** If your skin isn't too sensitive, use a chemical exfoliant (more on this on page 48). Alpha-hydroxy acids, such as lactic or glycolic acid, are gentler on the skin.

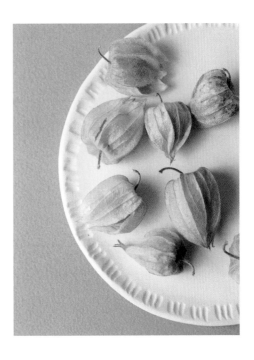

Beetroot lip and cheek balm

For: A nourishing lip treat that doubles as a make-up product. This lip tint not only beautifies – the shea butter nourishes your lips.

1 tablespoon shea butter
½–1 teaspoon beetroot (beet) powder
1 drop peppermint essential oil

If there was one make-up product I wouldn't go without, it's a lip and cheek tint. I'm all for a multipurpose product, especially when it has benefits for my skin. Lip and cheek tint is also the one product that I think transforms your whole face, giving you a youthful healthy glow. I've got about five lip and cheek tints strewn around my car and in my handbags. One of the good things about this balm is that you can adjust the amount of beetroot depending on how rich you want the colour. The other great thing about this little pot of beauty is that the ingredients melt into your skin, so it's easy to apply on your lips and cheeks.

To make: In a small saucepan over a very low heat, melt the shea butter.

Remove from the heat and gradually stir in small amounts of the beetroot powder whilst stirring until you're satisfied with the colour.

Stir in the peppermint essential oil.

Pour into a small container and let it cool and harden.

To use: Apply like a regular lip balm or dab it on your cheeks. Less is more with this product! The colour can build quite quickly.

Use as often as you like!

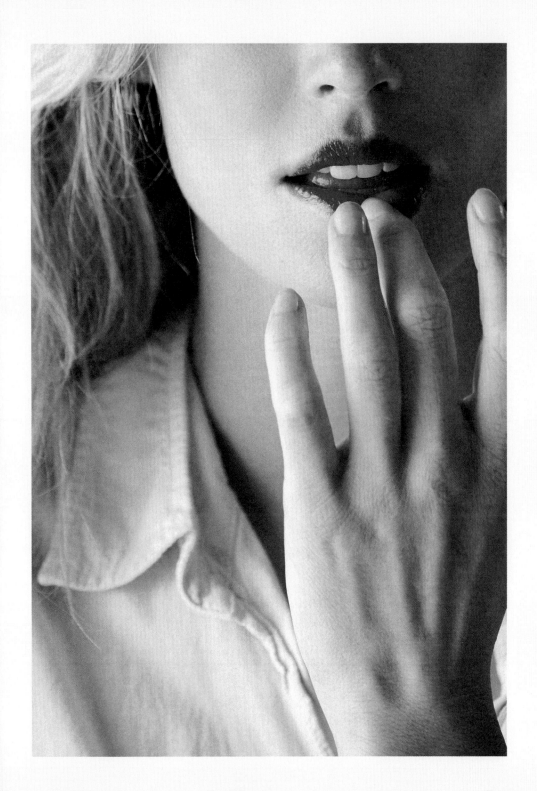

Exfoliants

The importance of exfoliation was one of the first things I learned about skincare. Exfoliating is key because when we have too much build-up on the stratum corneum, the outermost layer of skin, it can get overwhelmed, compromising its ability to do its job of keeping our skin protected and moisturised. It's not just the build-up of dead skin cells, but also pollution and oil that contribute to the gunk we might not be able to see with our naked eyes. You can imagine the work it must do to keep out the toxins and chemicals from today's polluted world. If your stratum corneum isn't happy, you'll start to see irritation, dryness, blotchiness and even infections. Exfoliating helps clean our skin and increase healthy skin cell turnover, thereby improving our skin barrier function.

Exfoliating can also help your pores. When your pores look enlarged, it can mean they're full of dead skin cells, oil and dirt. Chemical exfoliants, such as alpha-hydroxy acids or a fruit enzyme mask, will help minimise your pores, but a daily scrub with a washcloth and a good cleanser will prevent large pores. Start slow with exfoliation and look for signs of inflammation like redness. If you have sensitive skin, you'll need to be extra cautious, but there are still options for you too. It's always a good idea to make sure you protect your skin by adding a nourishing serum or oil after exfoliating, but you won't need to worry about this if you use a scrub that already contains oil.

A word of warning – don't exfoliate too much. In my opinion, we can get overly obsessed with acids and physical exfoliants when sometimes all that we need is a washcloth and a little cleanser. Over-exfoliating can inflame your skin, mess up its pH level and leave it vulnerable to environmental factors. Wearing sunscreen is important, but it's especially crucial when using a chemical exfoliant that can increase your skin's sensitivity to the sun.

....

Tips & Tricks: Everything we rub, spray or lather onto our skin can end up coming into contact with capillaries and veins and go right into our bloodstream. The lipid matrix in our skin is our friend, and lots of skin conditions happen when it's damaged. Focusing on what's going on here and just underneath the very top layer with supportive vitamins and oils is what lies at the core of my natural beauty creations.

Physical exfoliants

Physical exfoliants are things like scrubs (page 74), baking soda and even a washcloth. It's thought that salt scrubs have been used to exfoliate skin since the days of the ancient Greeks, and they have stood the test of time, being just as effective today.

Although scrubs can be used anywhere, you need to be extra careful when using them on your face. Choose a soft grain as opposed to larger sugar or salt granules. Scrubs made with smaller granules, like caster sugar or almond meal instead of brown sugar, are better if you want to use the scrub on your face.

I don't recommend face scrubs because of the risk of breaking capillaries. There are other ways to exfoliate your face. However – lips are the exception. I adore my lip scrubs. They remove dead skin, giving you smooth lips instantly, and they stop you from having to rely on your lip balm so much. They will resurface the skin on your lips and make lipstick application much easier. If you need to quickly prepare your lips for a smooth lipstick application, then just whip up some honey, caster sugar and a little oil together in a small bowl and apply to your lips. Rub your lips with the scrub, then rinse. If you want a little bit of a lip plump, add a drop of peppermint or cinnamon oil.

Chemical exfoliants

There are two types of acids that are used as chemical exfoliants: alpha-hydroxy acids (AHAs) and beta-hydroxy acids (BHAs). These acids occur naturally, like the ones found in fruits, while other more concentrated versions are produced in labs. I would always suggest going with natural to begin with, but I will give you both options.

AHAs are found in fruit enzymes and accelerate the skin's natural shedding process by getting rid of that annoying visible layer of dead skin on the epidermis whilst clearing out pores. My favourite AHA mask is a cranberry mask. It helps remove the dead skin that tends to appear after you use a retinoid product (page 53) without a physical exfoliant. AHAs, namely lactic and glycolic acids, are a milder choice than their cousin BHAs and are more suitable for dry or sensitive skin.

Caution! AHAs cause sensitivity to sun, so only use them at night and use sunscreen during the day. Often you can find AHA and BHAs in leave-on exfoliating face serums to use at night.

Lactic acid, a type of AHA, comes from beetroot (beet), sugarcane and cornstarch. It's most commonly made by fermenting these ingredients with lactobacillus bacteria (yes – a probiotic). Almost all lactic acid used is from these sources; however, a tiny portion may be derived from milk. Our body also creates lactic acid when we convert food into energy. Lactic acid is unique in that it not only exfoliates and cleans, but also moisturises. It stimulates the production of hyaluronic acid in our skin too. It's my favourite exfoliant and the acid I use when I have clogged pores or dry, flaky skin.

Glycolic acid, another AHA from sugarcane, has a slightly smaller molecular size, which allows it to penetrate slightly deeper than lactic acid, and is the highest potency AHA. Use it at a low concentration so your skin can get used to it; 2 to 5 per cent is plenty. I use this as a spot treatment for pimples.

BHAs are known as salicylic acid or betain salicylate. They are oil-soluble acids that are a little stronger and penetrate deeper than AHAs. They are only recommended for oily skin that has been exposed to other acids before, as it can be quite harsh or irritating. Salicylic acid is stronger than betaine salicylate and only needs to be at a concentration of 0.5 per cent to be effective.

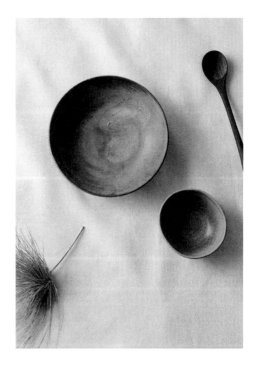

DIY natural microdermabrasion

For: Sloughing off dead skin cells and reducing scarring.

I can't say microdermabrasion is a treatment I have ever tried in a clinic. I have heard both good and bad things about it, although more recently I have heard it can be quite harsh and damaging to the skin, especially if you have somewhat sensitive skin. I'm all for a bit of exfoliation, but it's not necessary to head straight to the clinic when you can try this treatment at home.

2 teaspoons organic bicarbonate of soda (baking soda)
½–1 teaspoon lemon juice (depending on skin sensitivity)
½ teaspoon water

To make: Add all the ingredients to a small bowl and stir together thoroughly into a paste.

To use: Use a spatula or your fingers to massage the paste into your skin for about 5 minutes. Rinse your face, then moisturise and enjoy your fresh, smooth and glowing skin!

Use once a week or once every two weeks.

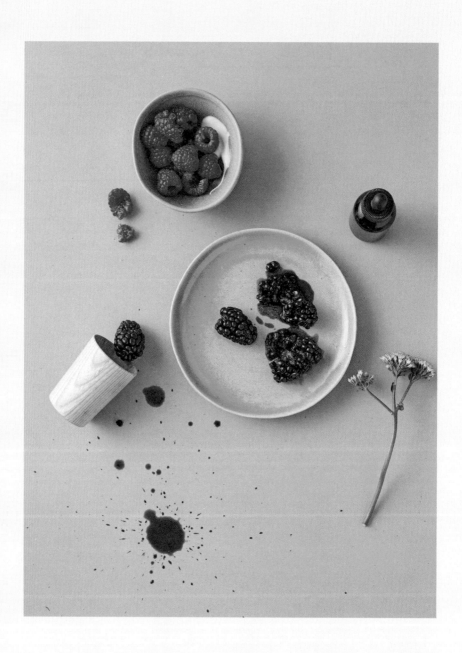

Berry enzyme mask

For: An extra exfoliating boost.

I'm always using berries for beauty. Not only are they great for our health and full of vitamin C, strawberries even whiten our teeth! I also love recipes that use up food that is no longer fresh enough to eat, as I hate waste.

The alpha-hydroxy acids in berries help exfoliate dead dry skin off your face, and the lactic acid in yoghurt supercharges this effect – you can use coconut or soy yoghurt for a vegan option. Lavender oil is really soothing for the skin, that's why I added it here – and, of course, it smells heavenly.

½ cup organic yoghurt
  or coconut yoghurt
  or soy yoghurt
¼ cup blueberries
¼ cup raspberries
1 drop lavender essential oil

To make: Blitz the yoghurt and berries together in a blender until the berries have broken down completely.

Pour the mixture into a bowl, add the lavender essential oil and stir to combine.

To use: Apply the mask to a clean face, neck and décolletage and leave on for 10 minutes. If you notice a little tingling, that's OK – it is the alpha-hydroxy acids working their magic.

Use once or twice a week.

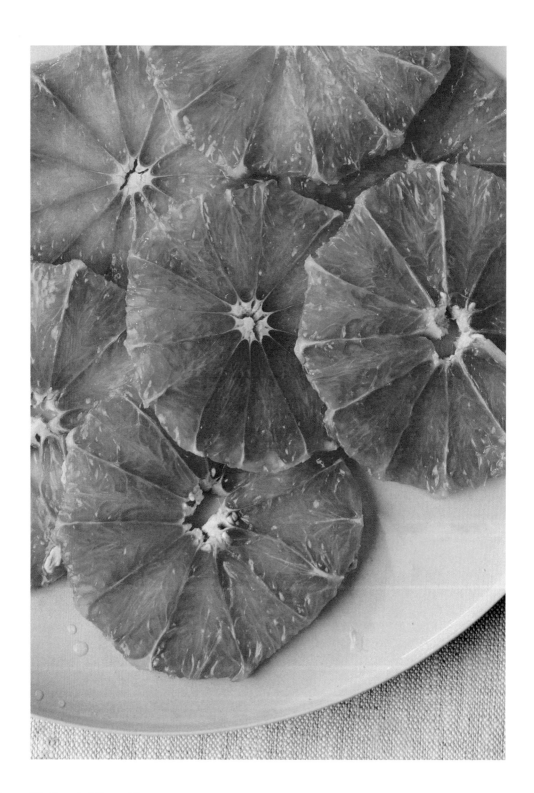

Topical vitamins: A, B and C

Vitamin A

First up: vitamin A. You've probably heard of beta-carotene. It's the orange pigment that makes carrots and pumpkin the colour they are. When we eat beta-carotene, it turns into vitamin A in our bodies, providing us with a strong antioxidant that helps with bone tissue and skin cell growth and repair.

Retinoids are derived from vitamin A and are used to treat acne, due to their ability to increase cell regeneration. This is where things can get a little more complicated. When retinoids are synthetically processed and made into a standalone ingredient, they can be quite irritating. You're more likely to have heard of retinol, a specific type of retinoid in over-the-counter cosmetics. Prescription retinoids are usually stronger than over-the-counter retinol products, but keep in mind that even retinol can cause sensitivity in some people. If you're pregnant or thinking of having a baby, retinol or retinoid use and supplementation is not recommended.

If you're using retinoid-based products, gradual use is necessary for your skin to get used to it. Don't freak out if your skin seems a little irritated – you'll just need to take it easy and slow. I recommend going with a low dose and not using it every night.

Avoid combining it with chemical exfoliants (page 48), because this will cause more irritation to your skin. However, products containing niacinamide (page 54) can help reduce some of the inflammation.

Personally, I don't use prescription retinoids at all because I feel the accumulative result of using gentler retinoid products, for example retinyl palmitate, every other day is effective enough. I don't tend to use retinol too often either, mainly because I find its skin-sloughing effect a little annoying. I feel that the focus should always be on whole plant–based ingredients, rather than trying to synthetically produce super-concentrated versions. However, in saying that, skincare ingredients like vitamin A are real powerhouses in helping our skin age at a rate that we are more comfortable with.

....

Tips & Tricks: Our skin can be more sensitive when we have our periods, so reduce your use of acids and retinoids during that time as they do have the potential to be irritating to the skin.

B vitamins

As for the Bs, there's actually eight different B vitamins. The one that's really changed my skin is vitamin B3, otherwise known as niacinamide or nicotinamide. Niacinamide is thought to help reduce hyperpigmentation and excessive wrinkles, as well as strengthen the skin's barrier. That's all good, but they're not the reasons why I use it. I find it really helps with inflammation. My skin naturally goes quite red, but when I apply a niacinamide cream at night, I don't wake up with the redness around my nose and chin that I otherwise would have. One of the best things about it is that it's great for any skin type, even if you suffer from conditions such as rosacea.

Vitamin C

You've no doubt heard of super-antioxidant vitamin C's usefulness for helping reduce cold and flu symptoms, but how about its skin benefits? Whether you're consuming it or applying it topically, vitamin C is a powerful antioxidant that can have a brightening, skin-perfecting effect. It's also great for reducing hyperpigmentation and free radical damage; it can help limit the formation of free radicals in skin caused by everything from UV rays to pollution.

Vitamin C even has a slight sun-protective effect. This should make it part of your morning skincare routine. It's the first serum I put on my skin before a thick moisturiser and my mineral sunscreen.

Vitamin C is often labelled as ascorbic acid in ingredient lists, or ascorbyl tetraisopalmitate in oil formulas. Vitamin C is more stable and less likely to become rancid in an oil product. Try to find an oil serum with vitamin C or a miracle Australian extract from Kakadu plums – the most potent natural source of vitamin C.

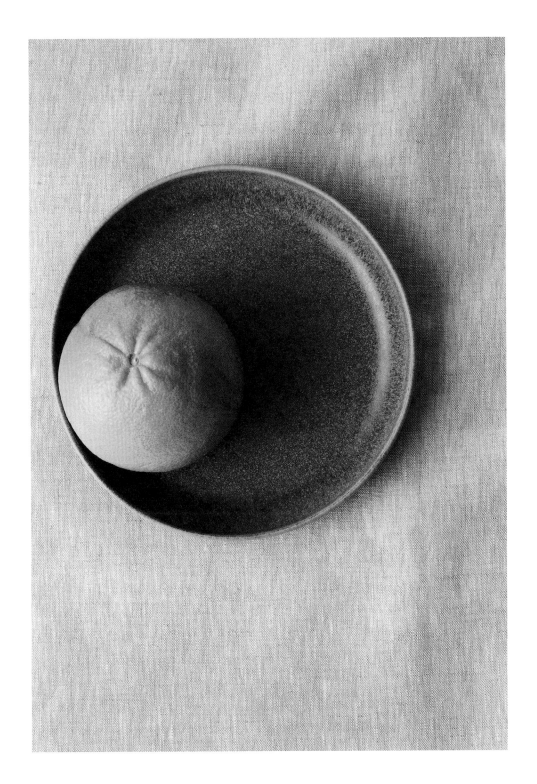

Gua sha

Have you seen those little rose quartz massage stones pop up on your social media? Or maybe the jade rollers? They both have a similar effect, but what exactly do they do? In a sentence, they are great for de-puffing your face, but that's not what they were originally made for. Gua sha is an ancient traditional Chinese medicine technique that has been used for centuries to stimulate our skin and lymphatic system. The traditional massage is *incredibly* painful. It involves scraping the sharp crystal all over your body, including places like your shin bones (ouch!), leaving you with bruises.

I personally would recommend using the smooth stone tools on the market now and taking a gentler approach, keeping it to your face where you can still stimulate your lymphatic system and release tension in your jaw – a much more palatable option to an all-over body torture. You can perform a gua sha facial ritual at night or in the morning, but I would recommend doing it in the morning to help remove any puffiness and get your lymphatic system moving. Quality matters when it comes to buying a gua sha or jade roller. Fake copies have flooded the market, and you want the real deal, so buy from a reputable supplier.

....

Tip: Keep your tool in the fridge for extra de-puffing benefits.

- You will need to apply a serum or oil to your skin first (apply to both your face and neck). Jojoba or rosehip oil are great options, and you can even use aloe vera.

- Holding the tool firmly, start by pressing it into the middle of your chin and move along your jaw line towards your ears. Repeat a few times. I like to focus on my jaw joint and use the pointy part of the tool to press in and release tension there.

- Then move the tool to the space above your top lip and press down lightly while moving it across the face towards your ear.

- Move up the face to your cheeks. Start from the part of the cheek that is closest to the nose and press out towards your ears. If you're stone isn't big enough, you can massage your top cheek first and then do the lower cheek after.

- For your nose, start between the brows and push down.

- Be extra gentle with your eye sockets. Push gently on the eye socket and brow bone area and push outwards.

- Move to your forehead. For your middle forehead, start between the brows and push upwards towards your hairline. For the sides, start from the centre and push outwards towards your hairline.

- Practise for a couple of minutes. If you use a jade roller instead of the rose quartz tool, the process is the same.

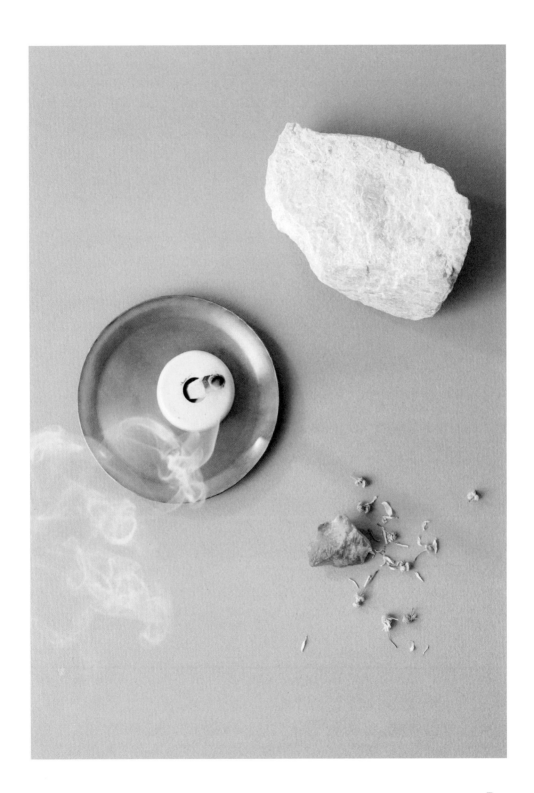

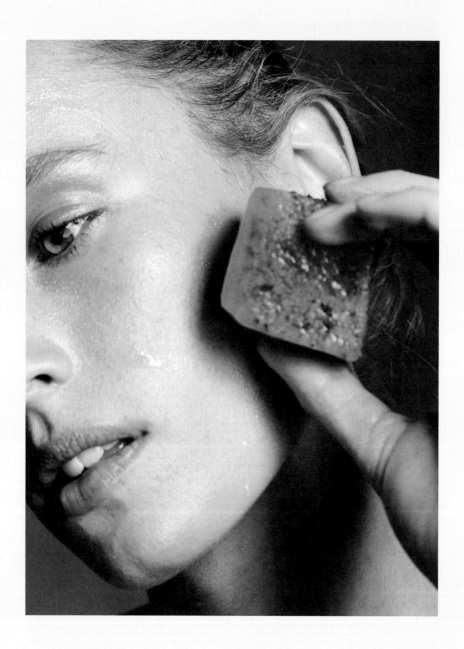

The Botanical Beauty Hunter

Cooling herbal ice cubes

For: Soothing a puffy face.

A great way to use herbs that are no longer good enough to eat is to make these herb-infused ice cubes to soothe your face and assist in de-puffing. They are a great antidote to a hangover and are total lifesavers on a hot summer's day. They work like mini cryotherapy for your face and act like an instant facial. You can use the frozen cubes on your face whenever you please, but after cleansing in the morning is my favourite time. For an instantly more nourishing facial, add a drop or two of plant oil on your face before you rub the ice block over. This is a celebrity facialist's trick and great to use just before an event to get extra glow.

1½ cups water
2 green tea bags
2 peppermint tea bags
1 cucumber (puréed)
2 teaspoons finely
  chopped mint
1 teaspoon finely
  chopped parsley
1 teaspoon finely
  chopped rosemary

To make: Boil the water in a saucepan.

Turn off the heat and add the tea bags. Steep for 10 minutes, then remove the bags.

Let the tea cool, then add the puréed cucumber.

Add the chopped herbs and stir to combine.

Fill an ice-cube tray, being careful to stir the water continuously as you pour to make sure you are getting herbs in each section of the tray, then freeze.

To use: Rub an ice cube gently over your face. You can let the residue sit for 5 minutes before wiping it off if you like.

Use as often as needed.

Eye care

The skin around our eyes requires different care from the rest of our face. It's important that face moisturisers are kept at least a quarter-inch away from the bottom lash line. The thin skin around our eyes has tiny pores and the eyelid skin should never have skincare products applied to it.

I learnt this the hard way when a few of those hard-to-get-rid-of white spots, called milia, appeared under and around my eyes. They were appearing because I was using my face moisturiser on that delicate under-eye skin. For the record, glycolic acid removed my milia overnight, but it's not recommended for use on the skin near your eyes.

Since then, I have always given special care to the skin around my eyes, as we all should. A light eye serum might be your best option, as petroleum-based and preservative-rich eye creams can also cause milia. Otherwise, a homemade cream without preservatives or synthetic fragrance can work a treat.

De-puffing

Drinking alcohol and eating delicious, rich foods, fluid retention, hormonal changes and allergies are the major reasons for our very unwelcome under-eye bags. Salt causes some people to retain water and look puffy, but the inflammation that sugar causes wreaks havoc (remember, there's also sugar in alcohol!). Genes play a role in terms of how your body reacts to things like sugar and alcohol. It's worth remembering that the best thing about consuming alcohol is usually the social

setting in which it's consumed, rather than the drink itself. Hangover face does not come with an easy cure unfortunately.

Preventing the water retention that causes eye puffiness can start with your morning tea. Consuming foods and drinks with a diuretic effect, such as dandelion tea, will not only prevent your eyes from becoming puffy, but your whole body. Back in the day, before a big photoshoot, I would always take a couple of herbal diuretics the night before to help eliminate puffiness. Celery and parsley are also diuretics, so add these to your salads.

I have found that when I take antihistamines for my hay fever, they also reduce puffiness in my face. Allergies and sensitivities, for instance to pollen or certain foods, can cause skin puffiness and eye bags, so taking an antihistamine before a big event might be a good idea.

There are a few tricks to help with eye bags and puffiness – for example, the Green tea ice cubes (page 66), gua sha (page 56) and placing green tea bags on your eyes – while you get to the root cause of your eye puffiness. Perhaps you have a hidden allergy to a food or even the feather pillows you sleep on, or maybe you just drink a few too many cocktails!

If you don't have the time for the Green tea ice cube eye treatment, make sure you have a mist spray bottle filled with green tea, mineral-rich water or a floral hydrosol next to your bed, so you can mist your face upon waking. Bonus points if you also keep an extra cold one in the fridge.

The green tea bag trick isn't an old wives' tale, either. The caffeine in a tea bag is likely much more than you'll find in any eye cream, and it's great for reducing puffiness as it acts as a diuretic, removing residual fluid. Just soak a couple of green teabags in room-temperature water for a couple of minutes, then chill them in the fridge. Close your eyes, place the cold tea bags on your eyelids and think good thoughts for about 10 minutes. (Obviously, the thinking part's not compulsory.)

Brightest whites

As for your actual eyeballs, we all want clear whites, as this is a sign of good health. If they are yellow, this can signal disease, so you'll want to see a doctor quick sticks. A former partner of mine always used to be jealous of the clear whites of my eyes. He would suffer from bloodshot eyes often and would come home looking like he'd spent the day fighting fires, the poor guy. At the time, I didn't know what could be causing it, but now I know it was likely a vitamin B2 deficiency, in which case I would have been suggesting he eat way more green vegetables and eggs.

If you're staring at a computer screen a lot, like I am while writing this wonderful book, then you might want to invest in some blue light–blocking glasses. The light from our devices can leave us wired and unable to sleep, and blue light–blocking glasses can help, as can a technology-free hour before bed. Ayurvedic tradition also advises against using hot water near our eyes and to instead opt for lukewarm water around our eyes and heads when we can. In terms of eating for eye health – the best eye-nourishing antioxidants are vegetables and fruits that are predominantly purple, so throw some blueberries in your smoothie and whack some purple cabbage in your salad.

Dark circles

Dark circles are caused by broken capillaries, which then attract enzymes that break down the red blood cells, turning them dark blue. It's the same way that bruises are caused, which is why arnica, traditionally a herbal treatment for bruises, can help correct dark circles.

When I started experimenting with DIY beauty and was looking for a treatment for the dark circles around my eyes, I placed a couple of raw potato slices just under my eyes. To be honest – I lasted all of 30 seconds before my boyfriend and I collapsed in laughter at my ridiculousness. There's method to my madness though; the enzyme in potato does work as a skin lightener, helping reduce dark circles.

I can promise you – the majority of the eye creams you buy are totally ineffective and not tailored to your needs, so DIY natural treatments win here. In the end, it's a bit of trial and error, as your circles and puffiness are caused by different things requiring different treatments.

Tips & Tricks: I swear by milk thistle tablets for dark circles. I don't take them all the time, but they work better than any eye cream ever could. Just take a few at night – they work overnight.

Removing eye make–up

To remove make-up from the delicate eye area, I can only implore you to use a plant oil. Once you try it, you won't go back. Oil on a cotton pad removes make-up instantly and, because it isn't harsh and slides easily on skin, it doesn't burst any of the delicate blood vessels surrounding your eyes. When you use plant oils around your eyes, be careful not to get it in your eyes like I seem to do every single time. (You'll just get a little bit of blurry vision for a minute before your eye gets rid of it naturally.) I don't recommend using undiluted essential oils around your eyes at all, even though some reputedly have benefits. I had a horrific experience when I put undiluted carrot seed oil under my eyes. Totally my own fault: I was testing to see if it would do anything for dark circles and didn't even think to mix it with a plant oil. After applying it, I took myself off to bed, only to feel like someone had rubbed chilli into my eye sockets a couple of minutes later. Not what you want!

Lead in cosmetics

Ancient Egyptians may have been the first to experiment with cosmetics, but they were also the first to use toxic ingredients. Their exaggerated eye make-up, which we still see today (in the form of thick, winged black eyeliner), contained ingredients such as malachite (a green copper), galena (lead sulfide) and soot. If you think times have changed and now we only use safe ingredients in make-up, then I'm afraid you're wrong. Lead, which has been associated with neurotoxicity, is still present in cosmetics. It's not even necessary for it to be labelled, as it's regarded as a contaminant and not an ingredient. Thank heavens we don't go around slathering white lead cream (or cerussa, the main ingredient in those once-popular lead paints) on our faces like the ancient Greeks did.

Coffee and arnica eye balm

For: Dark circles.

I've searched high and low for a magic eye cream. Turns out, it doesn't exist. I was left with no choice but to create my own.

The following ingredients are crucial for reducing and preventing that tired eye look. Arnica is traditionally used to reduce bruising, so naturally it can help with dark circles too. Carrot seed essential oil also reputedly helps with dark circles, but make sure it's always diluted. I've used sweet almond oil and evening primrose oil as diluents in this recipe, because they have dark circle reducing properties of their own. Caffeine helps reduce water retention and puffiness around your eyes.

¼ cup freshly ground
   coffee beans
¼ cup coconut oil
¼ cup beeswax
1 teaspoon evening primrose oil
1 teaspoon sweet almond oil
2 drops arnica essential oil
1 drop carrot seed essential oil
1 drop frankincense essential oil
1 vitamin E capsule or
   about 4 drops of vitamin E oil

Option: You can use the coffee grounds for a body scrub. Simply combine them with about 2 tablespoons of olive oil and a couple of drops of sweet orange essential oil.

To make: Create a DIY coffee strainer by putting a coffee filter in the opening of a wide-mouth mason jar. Fold the edges of the filter around the lip of the jar, then screw on the ring part of the jar to hold the filter in place.

Combine the coffee grounds and coconut oil in a small saucepan. Over a low heat, melt the oil and stir intermittently for 20 minutes, allowing the coffee grounds to slowly infuse into the oil.

Remove the mixture from the heat and pour it through the coffee strainer. Discard the coffee grounds (or use them for a body scrub, see option).

In another saucepan, melt the beeswax over a very low heat, and remove it from the heat as soon as it's melted. Add your freshly made coffee-infused oil, evening primrose oil, sweet almond oil and essential oils. Squeeze the vitamin E from the capsule into the mixture.

Mix thoroughly and keep in an airtight container, preferably in the fridge to keep the balm solid and for some extra de-puffing action.

To use: You can roll the balm in with a jade roller or just use your fingers.

Use nightly.

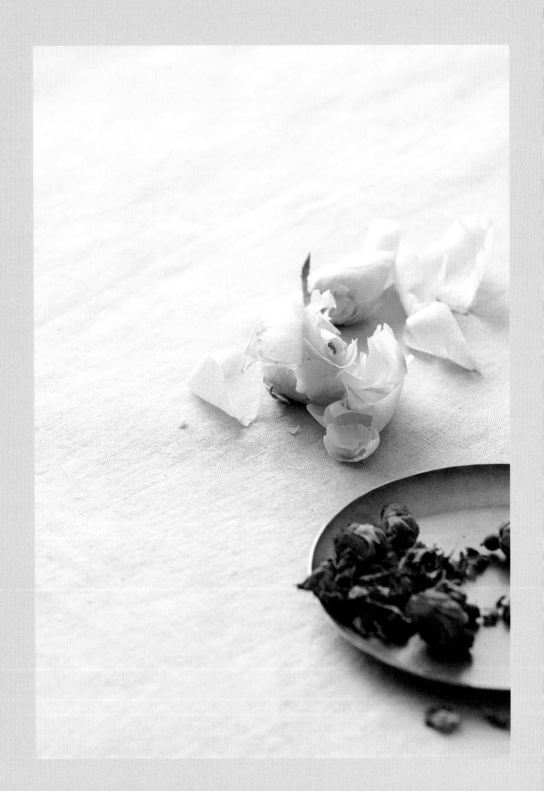

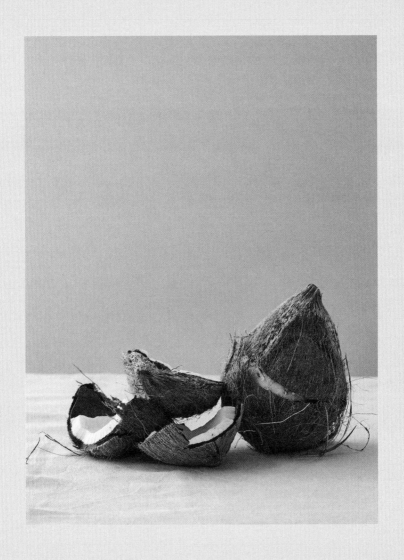

Green tea ice cube eye treatment

For: An instant wake-up treatment for tired eyes.

2 cups water
5 green tea bags

OK. You forgot to apply your eye serum before bed and you've woken up puffy. These little ice cubes will have an instantly revitalising and de-puffing effect, and they are extremely easy to make. I've really struggled to find effective eye creams, and sometimes simple is best. That's why I love these miracle cubes.

To make: Boil the water in a medium saucepan.

Turn off the heat. Add the tea bags and let them steep for 5 minutes.

Remove the tea bags and allow the liquid to cool.

Pour into an ice-cube tray and freeze.

To use: Gently rub the ice cubes over the skin under your eyes in a slow, outward motion.

Use as often as needed.

Lash growth serum

For: Longer, faster-growing lashes. This also works as a hair oil.

After many hours perfecting the hair oil treatment for my business, I've worked out that castor oil is a hair-saving wonder oil. It transformed my hair and helped it grow faster. It works wherever your hair is, so if you want fuller brows or lashes, you can use it there too – or anywhere else, for that matter! When used on lashes, castor oil will help your lashes regrow – and if you've gone through the hell of fake lash extensions, you'll find this serum extra beneficial. Your eye is the last place you want toxic chemicals, so I would always avoid lash extensions and focus on caring for the health of your existing lashes where you can.

1 tablespoon castor oil
1 tablespoon extra-virgin
  olive oil
1 vitamin E capsule or
  about 4 drops of vitamin E oil

To make: Combine the oils and the contents of the vitamin E capsule in a jar, stirring them thoroughly to mix.

To use: Shake the jar before use, then use a clean mascara wand to apply the oil from the very bottom of your lash line to the tip of your lashes.

If some of it gets in your eyes, don't worry. It won't sting or hurt you, but it might just make your eyesight blurry for a few seconds.

Leave it on overnight.

Use nightly for a month to see results.

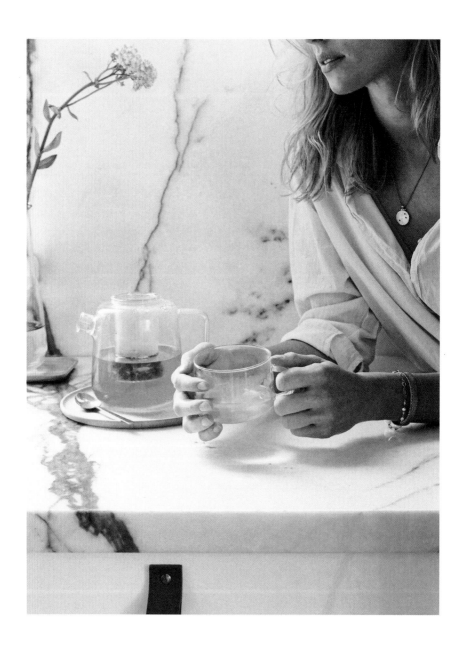

Tea

There are a couple of ways to use tea for natural beauty. Yes – drinking healthy herbal tea is one. The other is infusing tea in water to create facial steams. Tea quality matters. Generally, the larger the leaf, the better the quality. You'll also always want to go organic, because non-organic tea is often dusted with a concoction of chemicals.

I drink copious amounts of tea. I love it, and chances are, once you start, you will love it too. Tea can be a sacred practice. For me, it is one very obstinate part of my daily routine. I drink certain teas at certain times of the day, and I find they often replace snacking too.

You can start your day with a green tea if you insist on a little caffeine boost, although strong caffeinated teas can make some people feel a little ill on an empty stomach. I know that I will likely be sick if I have a strong green tea first thing, so I either make a weak one or just have a herbal variety, like gotu kola (or brahmi), a subtle-tasting herb with anti-anxiety properties, that is native to the wetlands of Asia. That herbal tea is on rotation for me at the moment. If you want to get serious health and antioxidant benefits, make a drink using the juice of a quarter lemon, some freshly grated ginger and some dried cloves in hot water, and drink it first thing in the morning.

White tea is another superstar tea, with an even higher amount of antioxidants than green tea. White tea actually contains more antioxidants than *any* other tea (aside from boiled cloves). There is research that shows white tea has anti-ageing effects, which include slowing the actions of the enzymes that break down collagen and elastin.

For skin that feels oily, some delicious licorice tea is your pick. Lucky you, licorice tea also helps stop sugar cravings. Some research shows the polyphenols in tea may reduce sebum secretion and acne, both when consumed and applied to the skin itself, so infuse it (pardon the pun!) into your life any way you can.

Rooibos, which comes from a shrub in Africa, is a major player in anti-ageing, with a plethora of antioxidants, zinc and even alpha-hydroxy acids. The zinc in rooibos tea can help correct the hormonal imbalances that trigger acne.

All teas contain antioxidants called catechins, along with an abundance of minerals and vitamins. Catechins are what you're after as they have been found to help with sun damage and premature ageing. In green tea varieties, epigallocatechin gallate is the most abundant catechin and is super potent.

....

Tips & Tricks: Herbal teas are known to be anticarcinogenic and help protect us against environmental damage. They can be quite heat sensitive; avoid using water above 70°C to make sure you don't burn away the tea's health benefits.

The polyphenols in green tea help prevent skin damage from sun exposure. L-theanine is another healthy amino acid found in green tea that is known to soothe and calm your skin. That's why green tea (in highly processed form) is now often added to skincare products. Usually these products also contain preservatives and palm oil derivatives, so your best option is to make your own fresh tea treatment at home.

Not keen on drinking tea? You can still reap the skin-loving benefits of tea by using it topically in your beauty routine. A green tea mist (just pour some cooled green tea into a mist spray bottle and voila!) upon waking or prior to applying a skin oil works an absolute treat in giving your skin a youth-boosting antioxidant bomb. There's also the toner on page 27, and then there are facial steams. For facial steams, you can chop and change as your heart (and skin) desires. Calendula and chamomile are your picks for sensitive skin. Sage and green tea are the duo for improved circulation and puffiness. Want to add some essential oils? Go for it! But only a drop or two so they don't get too overpowering. Eucalyptus, peppermint and rose are my favourites. Turn to page 17 for more on how to make your own facial steam treatment.

....

Tips & Tricks: While we're on the topic of facial steams, I have been known to keep a few eucalyptus leaves (OK, a small branch) in my shower so the oils infuse the room when the hot water hits them. If anyone uses your shower, they will think you have lost the plot trying to grow a tree in your shower, but it's worth it.

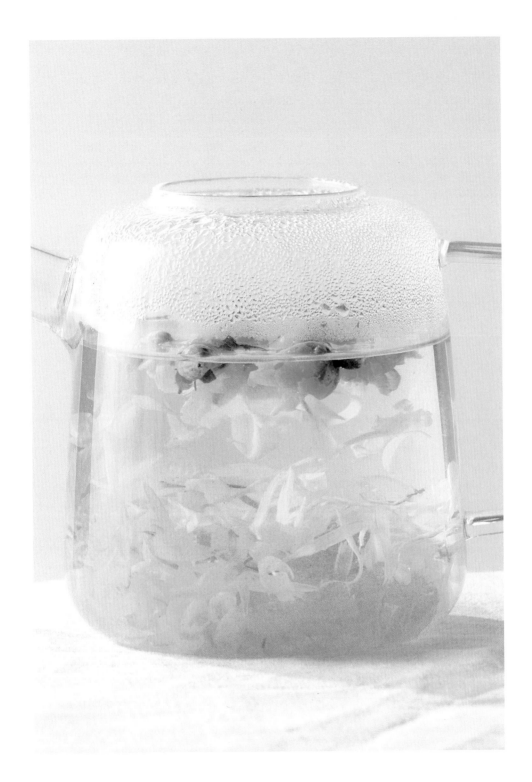

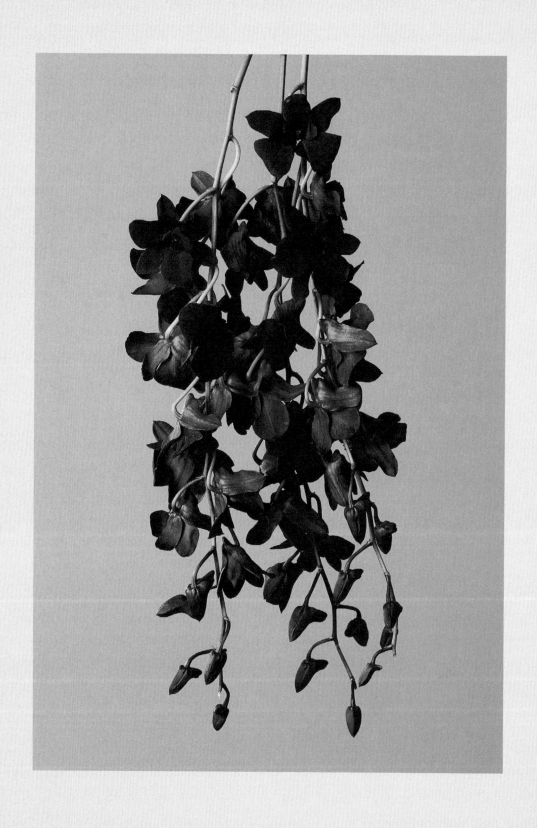

02

Body

I've often wondered why body products aren't given the same attention as face products. I personally think that my arms and legs love vitamins and nourishment just as much as my face does. Of course, caring for your body does take more time than just your face, but this time spent on yourself is priceless.

Our bodies respond so well to just a bit of care and love. I have included some self-care rituals in this chapter that not only benefit your skin and health, but also really allow you to connect with yourself. Practices such as self-massage and the inclusion of beneficial natural ingredients into your daily routine are major players in natural beauty, and also influence the way we feel about ourselves.

When was the last time you touched your body all the way from head to toe? I feel there's a sense of disconnect between ourselves and the miraculous flesh that we inhabit. When you think about it, our bodies and brains are amazing. A human can be renewing skin, carrying a baby, listening to music, digesting food and writing a book all at the same time. I want my body to be in the best condition possible to see me through my life, that's why taking care of it is so important to me.

Self-love is a stretch for some people, but simple daily or weekly practices that lend a connection with ourselves can get us on our way. I can say that lathering myself in a beautiful body oil, or having a soothing bath, can feel like a therapy session.

Scrubs

Physical exfoliants are very effective and best for regular use on your body, but be wary: if you're too harsh, you'll break capillaries, especially on sensitive skin.

Body scrubs are the easiest products to make at home, and are way cheaper to make than buy. As you can imagine, the way to make all body scrubs is pretty similar, and you probably have a lot of the ingredients in your kitchen already. Adjust the amount of oil depending on how you like it. Personally, I like to feel moisturised after I wash off my body scrub, so more oil is my preference. You might like a drier feeling – just have a play around. The recipes in this book contain enough mixture for a few uses, so make sure you have a spare waterproof container to keep them fresh for up to three months.

There are two times when you can apply a scrub. You can do it pre-shower on dry skin or in the shower. I find it easier to apply when I'm in the shower; my skin is warmer and the scrub seems to glide on much easier, but again, it's up to you, and the results aren't much different. Just make sure you get off all the bits in the shower (I always forget my shoulders!), otherwise you'll have to jump back in when you feel how sticky the back of your arms are.

AHA seaweed scrub

For: Skin needing a deeper exfoliation.

½ cup pink Himalayan salt
1 tablespoon apple juice
1 teaspoon powdered or
    crushed kelp
¼ teaspoon apple-cider vinegar

Since I grew up at the beach, I need a little bit of ocean in my beauty routine. Kelp is a nutritious iodine-filled seaweed that you can find at your Japanese grocer or online. It is mineral and antioxidant rich, and is known to help soften and hydrate dry skin. It reminds me of the smell of washed-up seaweed when playing on the beach as a child. The apple juice contains malic acid, a source of natural alpha-hydroxy acids. This scrub is great for oily skin, as the salt will get right into trouble spots and help clear them out.

To make: Combine all the ingredients in a bowl and mix thoroughly.

To use: Rub in a circular motion before your shower or in the shower (avoid being directly under the water).

Use three times a week.

Skin–softening and anti–inflammatory matcha and avocado oil scrub

For: Skin with free radical damage.

1 teaspoon matcha powder
½ cup coconut sugar
1½ tablespoons avocado oil
2 drops geranium essential oil

I first tried matcha at a tea ceremony in Japan and became a bit obsessed afterwards. It's not just great to drink – it has skin benefits when used topically. I have used it as an ingredient in face masks and body scrubs. I even have a matcha tea whisk that I use for tea ceremonies at home.

Matcha has been used for its antioxidant power, and it's also thought to be useful for reducing acne scars. Avocado oil is a beautiful softening and moistening plant oil that isn't too heavy. I use geranium essential oil almost every day on my skin and, along with carrot seed essential oil, it's a powerful anti-ageing tool.

To make: Mix the matcha powder and coconut sugar together in a bowl. Add the avocado oil and geranium essential oil and mix thoroughly.

To use: Rub in a circular motion before your shower or in the shower (avoid being directly under the water).

Use three times a week.

Brown sugar vanilla dessert scrub

For: Dry skin needing some TLC.

When I first tried this recipe I was only about nineteen, but it's stood the test of time and has remained one of my favourites. The smell is out of control, and you'll want to eat it right out of the jar. It smells like a mouth-watering dessert – you'll feel absolutely scrumptious afterwards. You can add a ½ teaspoon of ground cinnamon for a warming effect if you're using it in winter.

1 vanilla bean
1 cup brown sugar
⅓ cup melted coconut oil
⅓ cup honey

To make: Scrape the seeds from the vanilla bean and add them to a bowl along with the remaining ingredients. Mix thoroughly.

To use: Rub in a circular motion before your shower or in the shower (avoid being directly under the water).

Use three times a week.

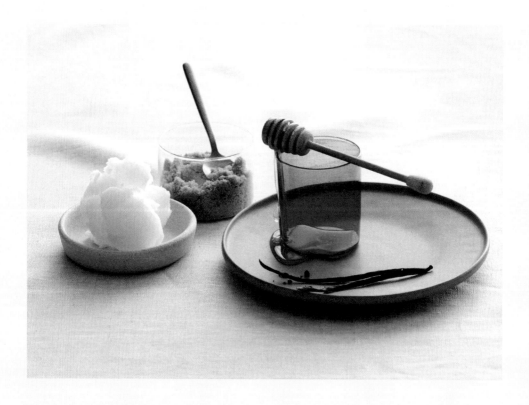

Herby freshening cucumber scrub

The herby nature of this scrub gives it a summer garden vibe and it is great to use in the morning. You can add a squeeze of lime to give it a cocktail feel.

For: Oily skin that needs energising.

½–1 small cucumber, chopped
1 small bunch of mint
1 small bunch of thyme,
  leaves picked
1 cup Himalayan pink salt
3 drops eucalyptus oil

To make: Blend the cucumber, mint and thyme leaves into a smooth mixture. Pour the mixture out into a bowl, then add the remaining ingredients and combine.

To use: Rub in a circular motion before your shower or in the shower (avoid being directly under the water).

Use three times a week.

Margarita scrub

This scrub has the added benefit of the naturally antiseptic tequila and lime, hence its ability to cleanse clogged pores. The tequila might make you feel a little strange if you use it in the morning, so it's best reserved for night showers.

For: Clogged pores and oily skin.

1 cup Himalayan pink salt
2 tablespoons melted coconut oil
  or sweet almond oil
1½ tablespoons tequila
grated zest and juice of 1 lime

To make: Combine all the ingredients in a bowl and mix thoroughly.

To use: Rub in a circular motion before your shower or in the shower (avoid being directly under the water).

Use twice a week.

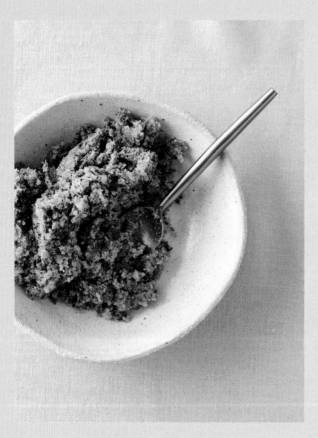

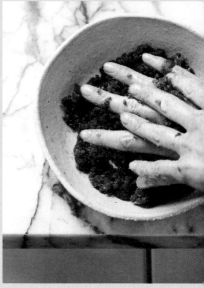

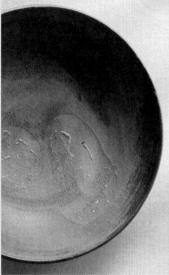

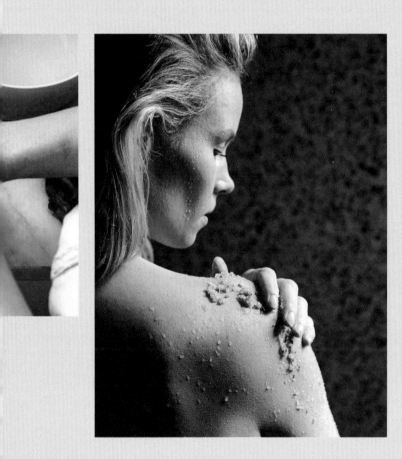

Cellulite

If you're like most women, you have cellulite. I've seen cellulite and stretch marks on the world's most famous supermodels, so don't feel like you're an outlier if you have it, especially if you're female. Oestrogen makes our skin differ from that of our male counterparts. The first-known use of the word cellulite appeared in 1873 in a French medical dictionary, where it was defined as the inflammation of the cell tissue. The term has only had a negative connotation since the 1980s.

So what is cellulite? When fat pushes through the fibrous netting that connects skin to muscle, it creates the dimple effect. Although it is common, cellulite can be exacerbated by a variety of things, including hormones, genetics, poor circulation or excessive alcohol consumption. Cellulite can be caused by the hormone-mimicking chemicals often found in conventional cosmetics – another reason to switch to natural. Parabens disrupt our hormones by mimicking oestrogen. Too much oestrogen can trigger cell division and tumour growth, which is why parabens have been linked to reproductive issues and breast cancer.

Although there is no magic cure for cellulite, there are things you can do to reduce it if you choose to. If I were you, I wouldn't bother trying too many in-clinic options. I have tried those machines that suck and push at your skin. You walk out after half an hour feeling a little red and bruised, without any miracle results to speak of.

Reducing cellulite is about diet, exercise and the products you use. The most effective things I've done was to consume less sugar and alcohol, and drink more water. I'm not the only one – upping water intake is one of the things that models do to prepare for photoshoots, along with avoiding salt. Herbs, teas and foods with a diuretic effect, such as celery and green tea, can help reduce puffiness in your body and have traditionally been used to reduce cellulite.

Essential oils diluted in a plant oil can help move fluid, reduce puffiness and stimulate the skin. My essential oil concoction for reducing cellulite and water retention is a secret recipe that us models used to use the night before shoots or fashion shows. It has the same essential oils – grapefruit and fennel – as my Anti-cellulite scrub (page 82). While essential oils help, don't forget you'll also want to be drinking at least 2 litres (68 fl oz) of water per day, including any herbal teas that take your fancy (preferably lymphatic-moving herb teas, such as nettle, burdock and dandelion leaf).

A relatively hard-core exercise program can get you results in as little as a month. A yoga class twice a week just ain't going to cut it, unfortunately. It's important to keep the circulation moving to reduce cellulite, and a firm massage can be a great help. Foam rolling, which can be torturous on sore muscles, can work wonders on cellulite. Lymphatic drainage massages work to keep everything moving in your body and help reduce water retention and toxins. Likewise, dry brushing (page 85) on the areas where you feel you have excess cellulite can help.

Stretch marks

Stretch marks are another stubborn friend you'll likely find appearing during puberty. They are the result of a loss of elastic tissue and collagen due to (somewhat obviously) skin stretching. Our genetics contribute to whether we get stretch marks, as does weight gain. Mostly, stretch marks show that you just, well, grew. Want to swap your stretch marks for being the size you were when you were eleven? Didn't think so. While the colour of stretch marks is easier to treat than the texture, both can be difficult. Body scrubs (page 74) can help by nourishing the skin and improving its texture, but it's pretty much impossible to rebuild the collagen. There are laser treatments, but I won't lie: you'll be paying a premium for little to no results. In my opinion, it just isn't worth it.

Here's a truth bomb: nobody notices your stretch marks like you do. It's like that with lots of things we are sensitive about. Truth is, very few people notice when you shave your legs, and even less your bikini line. The pimple on your chin? Didn't even glance at it. Us humans are so damn good at getting stuck in our heads, we forget about the compassion we actually have for those around us. If someone speaks ill of your stretch marks or cellulite, shame on them. I'd hate to think about the scrutiny they put themselves through.

Thank god for the body neutrality and body positivity movements for helping women realise that stretch marks and cellulite are not actual medical conditions and aren't things that need to be completely removed from our bodies. Don't sweat it. Most women have cellulite and stretch marks. You can definitely do things to reduce their appearance, but please don't waste your precious time, energy and brainpower on trying to remove them if you are already leading a healthy lifestyle. Our bodies are incredible, so try and focus on the miraculous tasks they are completing throughout the day without you even asking.

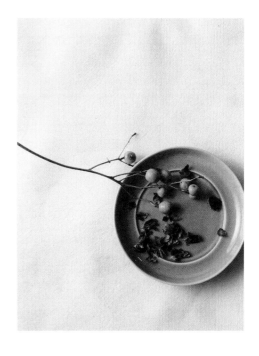

Anti-cellulite scrub

For: Reducing cellulite and improving circulation.

This scrub smells amazing! My anti-cellulite essential oil recipe is a secret, but it contains similar essential oils to the ones in this scrub. The ginger and essential oils help reduce cellulite and water retention. These essential oils have a revitalising effect, so this citrusy scrub is great for your morning shower.

1 cup brown sugar

2 tablespoons melted coconut oil or another oil of your choice

2 tablespoons freshly grated ginger

grated zest and juice of ½ lemon

6 drops grapefruit essential oil

2–4 drops fennel essential oil

To make: Combine the brown sugar and melted coconut oil in a bowl.

Add the grated ginger and lemon zest and juice and stir.

Add the essential oils and mix thoroughly.

To use: Rub on your desired areas in a circular motion before your shower or in the shower (avoid being directly under the water).

Use three times a week.

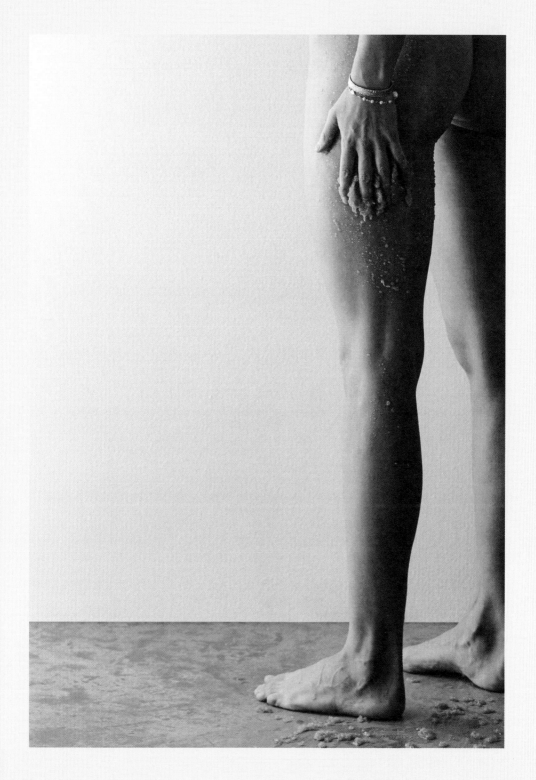

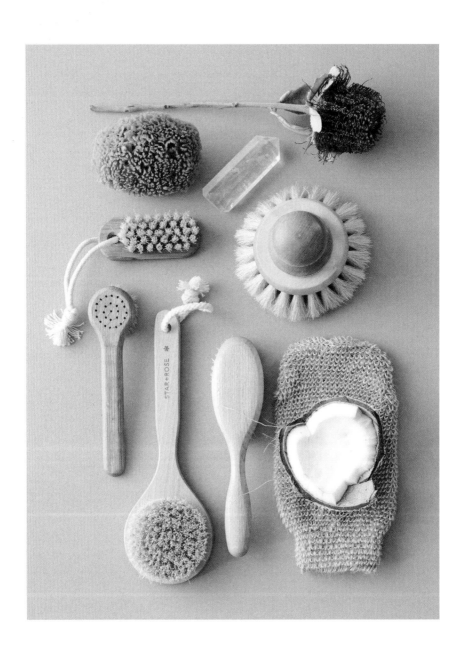

Dry brushing

Dry brushing is one practice that instantly makes your skin feel like you've had a spa treatment. Smooth, fresh skin is only seconds away.

Like body scrubs (page 74), dry brushing stimulates our lymphatic system and circulation, helping transport white blood cells, which help rid toxins from the body. It's nothing new: dry brushing was practiced in ancient Greece, and continues to be used to this day due to its effectiveness.

For me, it's the only thing that removes those really stubborn dead skin cells, like the ones on the back of my legs. Dry brushing is great for the blocked pores that can form on the back of your arms (keratosis pilaris). I have even heard of it being used for ingrown hairs, although I can't say I have tried this myself. It's going to feel a little uncomfortable at first if you're not used to it, because the brushes can be a little scratchy.

To dry brush, you'll need a special brush or an exfoliating mitt. There are plenty of bristle ones with wooden handles that allow you to scrub in all the right places. Just make sure you choose one that is made of natural materials, such as sisal fibres.

If you want, you can soften the blow by combing the brush with some body oil, such as rosehip or grapeseed. (Some brushes are made to be used with oil.) It will give you a little extra glide. Otherwise, apply body oil to your skin after brushing.

When we body brush, we always aim to be brushing towards our heart, except when we brush our stomach. I would never brush at night, as I find it too stimulating, but I'll leave that up to you to decide. If you have extra-dry skin, you can brush before your shower and wash the impurities down the drain, then apply a body oil straight after your shower.

Once or twice a week is plenty, and be gentle with yourself! We don't want to go around bursting capillaries.

I have a great mitt from Germany that I can just pop in the wash after using. Exfoliating mitts are easy to travel with and, *I swear*, are a jet lag cure sent from heaven. Nothing perks you up like a full body exfoliation after a flight! It's a great way to get our systems going again when we have been sitting on a plane not moving. It will help your blood flow, reduce water retention and, because of the lymphatic stimulation, you'll help rid your body of all the toxins it's collected from the aeroplane food and re-circulated air!

....

Tips & Tricks: Both scrubs and dry brushing exfoliate the skin, but using body scrubs will give you the benefit of extra moisturising because of their nourishing plant oils. I like to dry brush if I don't feel like I need the extra moisturising.

HOW TO DRY BRUSH

- Start at your feet (brush the top and bottom), then move with long strokes all the way up your leg, towards your heart. You'll want to do your whole leg, so don't forget the back.

- Move up to your bottom and brush up both sides towards your heart.

- Then move up to your stomach and brush in a clockwise direction.

- If you'd like to brush your back, make sure you pick a brush with a long handle.

- For your arms, start from your fingertips and move all the way past your elbows and to your shoulders. If you want to brush under your arms, and you're not ticklish, you can – just be extra gentle.

- For your chest, you should also be gentle as capillaries often lie close to the surface of the skin here. Massage this area from the middle of the chest outward in all directions.

- How do you feel? Energised? Smooth? Great! Stop here: don't even think about doing your face or neck, because the bristles will be way too harsh for these areas.

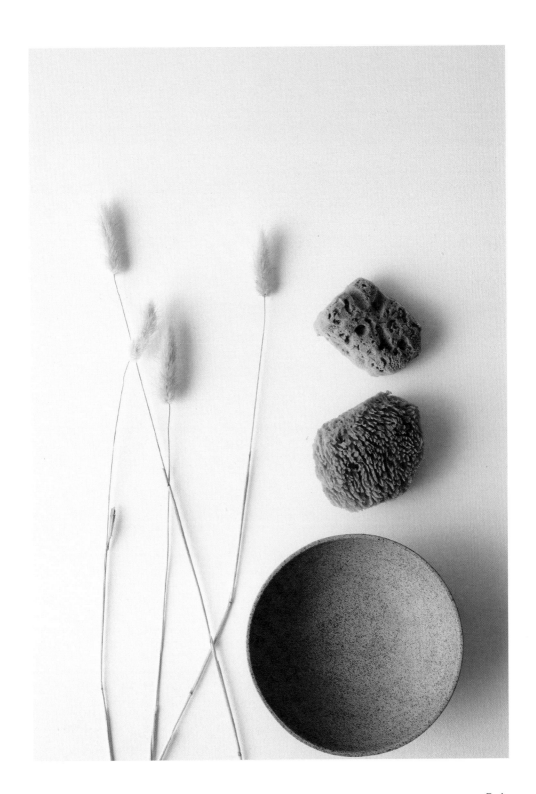

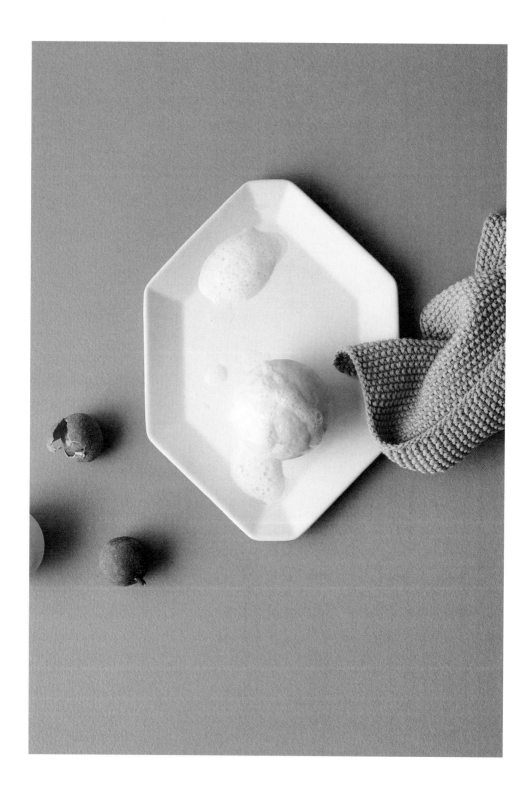

Bathing

I am an absolute bathing *fiend*. I'm not lucky enough to have a bath where I'm living now, so when I travel, it's always a luxury when my accommodation has one. One of my favourite travel memories is bathing in a traditional Japanese onsen, or hot spring, on a ski trip a couple of years ago. Thanks to its volcanic landscape, Japan has plenty of onsens sprinkled throughout the country, and they are absolutely beautiful. There are two things to note about onsens: you can't use them if you have tattoos, and you must be totally nude. I've got to say – nothing compares to swimming in a natural hot spring while snow falls. It's something I'll never forget.

I try my best to make my baths a sacred experience. The truth is – you don't need much. You'll find lots of ingredients in your pantry and fridge that can be used in baths. Rosewater, coconut milk, apple-cider vinegar and tea can all make your bath that little bit extra. There are plenty of bathing recipes that make you feel like you're in a day spa without having to leave your house. The recipes in this book have beauty benefits as well, so you'll look *and* feel your best afterwards.

Obviously, baths are relaxing. As our blood vessels dilate from the warm water, our blood pressure drops and our tensions melt away. There's nothing quite like that feeling of being submerged in a bath with your head underwater, is there? And if we add flowers, herbs and other nourishing plant-based ingredients, our baths can also have a medicinal effect. There's no need for synthetic fragrance–bubble baths or bath bombs full of skin-drying chemicals.

Oils are my favourite thing to add to baths – not just essential oils but also plant oils. These oils are important, because hot water can strip natural moisturising oils from our skin. Although I haven't experienced any plumbing disasters firsthand, oils can block drains, so don't add too much. A teaspoon will be enough; you can always put more directly on your skin afterwards. Also, be careful of slippery surfaces when getting in and out!

Lavender, chamomile and rose are the safest essential oils to add to a bath … *or* just use fresh flowers. For example, once when I had some roses that started losing all their petals, I scooped them up and sprinkled them in my bath. Roses are soothing and clarifying, and make me feel like a romantic goddess.

The Sanskrit word for bathing is snanam, which has connotations of spiritual cleansing. If you'd like an Ayurvedic approach, a self-massage with oil would precede the bath. Bathing isn't strictly related to your traditional baths either, especially in the Ayurvedic tradition. Bathing in clean rivers and lakes is just as (if not more) effective, if you're lucky enough to get the opportunity.

Vegan milk bath

For: Super soft skin.

We've all heard about the ancient beauty secret of milk baths. Most recipes call for cream and cow's milk. I personally wouldn't feel comfortable bathing in dairy, but coconut milk? Yes, please! It smells heavenly and has the same skin-softening benefits of regular milk.

1 vanilla bean
1½ cups full-fat organic
  coconut milk
¼ cup honey

To make: Scrape the seeds from the vanilla bean and combine them with the coconut milk and honey in a mixing bowl.

To use: Add to your bath and soak for 30 minutes or so.

Use as often as you'd like.

Detox bath

For: Sore muscles and skin in need of a deep clean.

Sometimes you just want to feel squeaky clean. This bath recipe will do that for you, along with giving you the healing and antioxidant benefits of clays, tea and oils.

1 cup Himalayan pink salt
1 tablespoon rhassoul mud
1 tablespoon bentonite clay
1 tablespoon kelp powder
1 tablespoon matcha powder
2 teaspoons vitamin E oil
5 drops rosemary essential oil
5 drops grapefruit essential oil

To make: Add all the dry ingredients to a bowl and stir to combine.

Add the vitamin E and essential oils and stir again.

To use: Add to your bath and soak for at least 20 minutes to get the full benefits.

Use as often as you'd like.

Tips & Tricks: It's recommended to bath two hours after eating, not immediately after.

Fizzy tangy bath powder

For: An energising bath experience.

½ cup bicarbonate of
    soda (baking soda)
½ cup citric acid
1 teaspoon grated orange zest
1 teaspoon grated lemon zest

I've always loved bath bombs, but they are just a bit too much effort for me to make for myself. This bath powder gives the fizzy fun part without having to spend hours crafting the perfect round shape.

To make: Mix the two powders in a bowl.

Add the orange and lemon zest and combine.

To use: Add to your bath. The more you add, the more fizz, so start with about one tablespoon before you add more.

Use as often as you'd like.

Antioxidant bath tea

For: Skin that is after a soothing antioxidant treatment.

½ cup Epsom salt
1 tablespoon dried
    calendula flowers
1 tablespoon white or jasmine
    tea leaves
2 teaspoons matcha powder
3 drops lavender essential oil

Option: If you don't have a bath, have a foot bath instead. Simply add the mixture to a container or bucket big enough for your feet and let it infuse into hot water.

I'm a huge fan of drinking tea and the herbs have a medicinal effect, so why not add them to your bath too?

I've made the mistake of adding copious amounts of tea to my bath without putting it in a teabag first, making the clean-up quite the task. You can use disposable or reusable tea bags here. You might find that reusable cotton muslin bags are more accessible than the disposable bags, which look a bit like coffee filters.

To make: In a bowl, combine all the ingredients except the lavender essential oil.

Add the lavender essential oil, stir and let it sit for about 30 seconds. Pour the mixture into a tea bag.

To use: Add the tea bag to your bath and let the ingredients infuse into the water before you step in.

Use as often as you'd like.

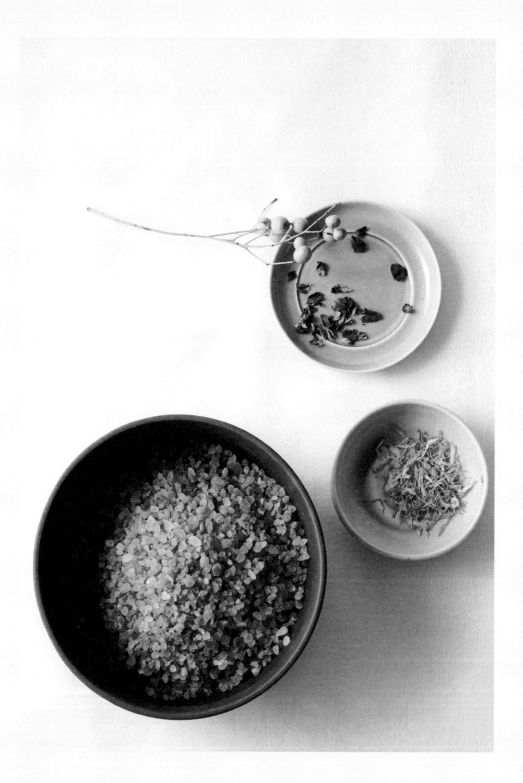

Ultimate flower bath salts

For: An instant detox that also helps with water retention.

I'll always vouch for the benefits of a Himalayan salt bath. It has a wonderful detoxing effect on the body and skin. I must say, though, it can get a little boring. That's why this recipe calls for flowers. It totally transforms the experience and makes me feel a bit like a fairy goddess, if I'm being honest. You need a lot of salt to really get the benefits here – this recipe makes enough for just one bath – so I recommend shopping at a bulk ingredient or health store, where you can pick things up relatively cheaply. As for the flowers, you can use fresh or dried, or a combination of both. This is my favourite thing to do with a bunch of flowers that aren't quite good enough to sit in a vase anymore.

3½ cups pink Himalayan salt
1 cup marigold petals
1 cup rose petals
1 cup lavender flowers

Option: If you have any favourite fragrant flowers, you can add them too!

To make: If you're using dried flowers, mix the salt and flowers together with your hands, bruising the flowers and allowing the salt to be infused by their aroma. Add the mixture to the bath as you fill it.

If you're using fresh flowers, add the salt to the bath as you are filling it and sprinkle the flowers on top of the water after it's filled.

To use: Hop in your bath and enjoy for at least 20 minutes.

Use as often as you'd like.

Skin-soothing bath and shower pouch

For: Irritated skin.

Bicarb soda (baking soda) is actually great to use if you suffer from eczema or skin disorders as it has the ability to help balance the pH level of your skin. Oatmeal is finely ground oats and helps soothe irritated skin, and the floral ingredients and essential oils will help calm inflamed skin. If you don't have a bath for this, then it's not a problem. Use it in the shower by rubbing it gently over your body under running water.

¼ cup oatmeal

¼ cup bicarbonate of soda (baking soda)

3 tablespoons dried calendula flowers or tea leaves

3 tablespoons dried chamomile flowers or tea leaves

2 tablespoon dried lavender flowers or 3 drops lavender essential oil

1 cotton muslin pouch or reusable nut milk bag

To make: Mix all the ingredients together and add them to the pouch (you might need a few pouches depending on their size). If you're using lavender essential oil, don't add it to the pouch; wait until your bath is full before adding the oil.

To use: Add it to the bath as you're filling up to brew a nice infusion. If you're using lavender essential oil, you can add this now.

You can leave your pouch in the bath or remove it after 10 minutes or so, or use it in the shower.

Use as often as needed.

Tips & Tricks: Don't forget about the ambience of your bathroom – it adds to the experience! Candles and music can do wonders.

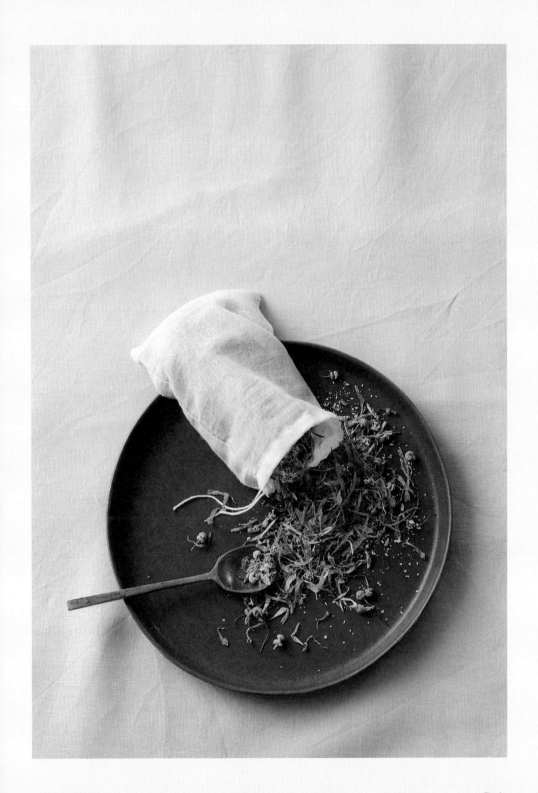

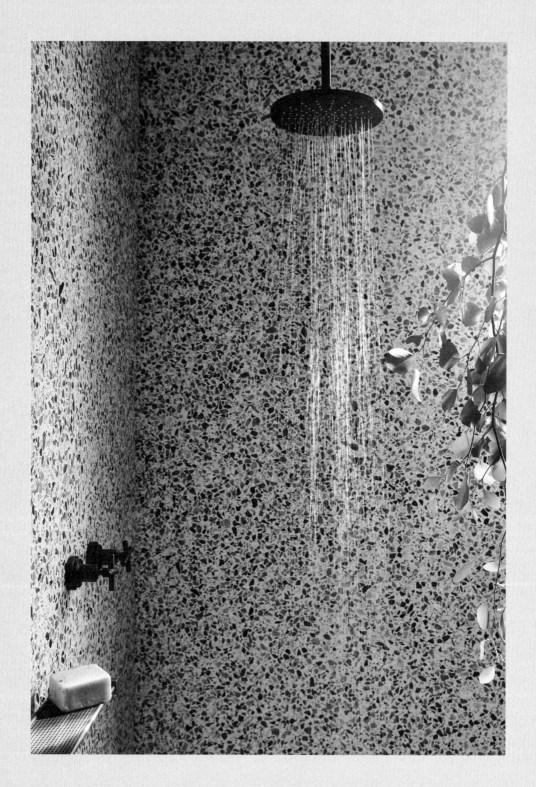

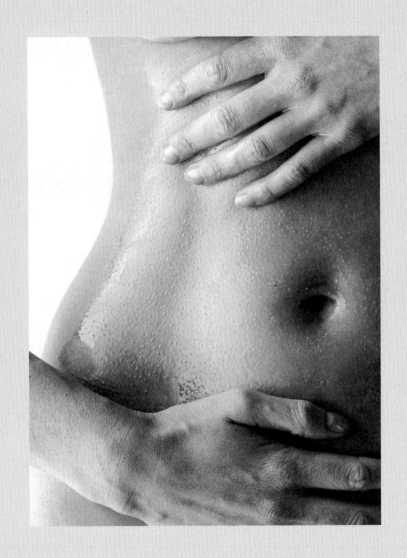

Bath melts

For: Skin needing extra nourishment.

These bath melts give you a nourishing alternative to conventional body moisturisers, and they smell divine. You'll get 10 bath melts from this recipe, so if you prefer less, then just halve the amounts.

There are two variations for scent with this recipe. You can either go with a rose–vanilla scent or opt for the sensitive skin alternative with lavender and oats.

2 tablespoons dried rose petals
1 vanilla bean (chopped
   into small sections)
½ cup shea butter
2 drops rose essential oil

To make: Grind the rose petals and vanilla bean together in a mortar and pestle to create a fine powder. Alternatively, you could use a coffee grinder.

Melt the shea butter in a saucepan over a very low heat while stirring in the rose and vanilla powder.

Sensitive or irritated skin option: Substitute the rose petals with lavender flowers and the vanilla bean with 1 tablespoon of rolled (porridge) oats, and use lavender essential oil instead.

Remove from the heat as soon as it's melted and combined, and stir in the rose essential oil.

Pour into small silicone moulds and let them set in the fridge or freezer. Once set, remove from the moulds and store in a container in your fridge.

To use: Place one bath melt in the water as the tub is filling up. Feel free to rub the bath melt over your body if it hasn't melted by the time you get in the bath.

Use as often as you'd like.

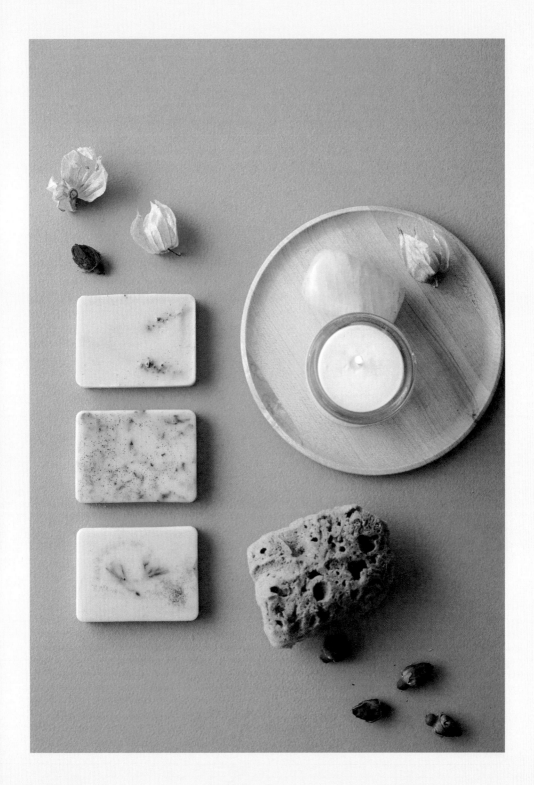

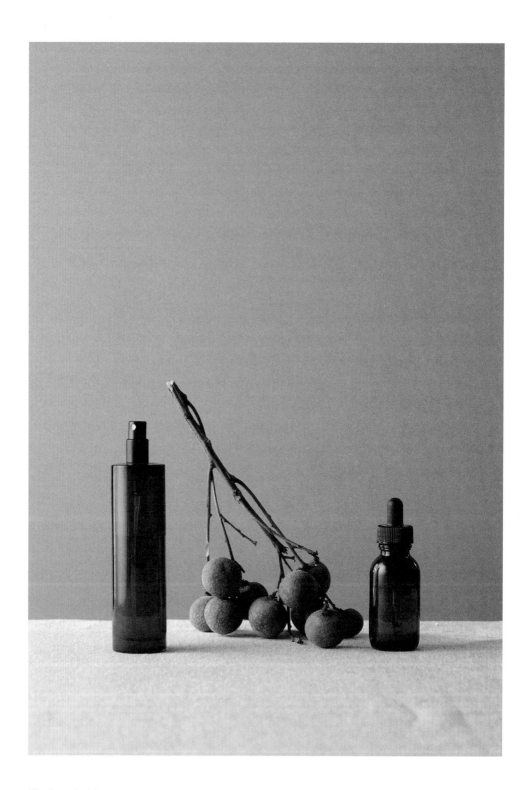

Oils, waxes and butters

You've got your creams – and you've got your oils. I'm going to preface this by stating that mineral oil (a.k.a. paraffin oil) is to be avoided like the plague. Mineral oil is a liquid by-product of refining crude oil to make gasoline and other petroleum products. The fact that this is what baby oil is made from makes me sigh out loud.

Conventional moisturisers contain water in their ingredients, and oils – obviously – don't. The water in cosmetics can be there for a couple of reasons, either to help the ingredients combine and help your skin absorb the moisturiser, or (more likely) to fill the product out and make it cheaper to manufacture. The major downside is that as soon as water is added to a cosmetic, companies need to add lots of potentially toxic preservatives to stop microbial growth.

Plant oils

First up, let me dispel the confusion between a plant oil and an essential oil. Plant oils, such as jojoba or rosehip, are fatty, non-volatile (non-evaporative) and not strongly scented plant extracts. Essential oils are natural, scented chemical compounds from fruits, flowers and barks. Plants generate them for a few reasons, such as assisting with pollination. Essential oils are known as volatile oils, meaning they evaporate at certain temperatures or under pressure. Direct application of undiluted essential oils onto the skin is not recommended, whereas plant oils can be used directly and liberally.

5 benefits of plant oils

1. They're multipurpose. You can use them all over your body, hair, scalp, in your bath, on your baby and even in the bedroom (coconut oil is an effective lubricant, although it isn't safe for use with condoms).

2. They give instant results. Most plant oils already naturally contain compounds such as antioxidants, polyphenols and omega fatty acids. These work straight away to change the appearance and texture of your skin, while also having the long-term effect of helping reverse skin damage.

3. They feel amazing. Synthetic and mineral oils are comedogenic (meaning they clog pores), while most natural plant oils are not (coconut oil being the big exception). Oils have a naturally nourishing, skin-comforting texture without the toxic silicones found in moisturisers.

4. Plant oils are relatively inexpensive. I stock up on oil and buy in bulk – choose cold-pressed oils if you can.

5. They work well together. You can make your own recipe tailored for your skin type and even add essential oils.

Plant oils have more than just the effect of making your skin feel soft and hydrated; they feed your skin with vitamins and minerals. These oils have the unique ability to deeply penetrate and nourish the dermis so it maintains its elasticity, hydration and strength. The best thing about plant oils is that they suit all skin types and are versatile; this is why they are my number one natural beauty ingredient and remedy.

There are three types of oil: unrefined, partially refined and fully refined. Unrefined oil or cold-pressed oil is often your most expensive option – the oil is simply filtered to remove unwanted material and not heated. This type of oil will have the most authentic smell, colour and taste, and will often be the most nutrient-rich option. It's your blue-ribbon choice of oil that you'll get the most benefits from. Partially refined oils are less common and can mean the oil has been deodorised or bleached with clay or charcoal. Fully refined oil is your filtered and naturally bleached option. If you want your coconut oil without the flavour, this is the option you would go for. Because refining an oil removes lots of its curative compounds, I would recommend choosing unrefined if you can.

A word of warning with oils: be careful where you apply them! The carpet in my bedroom is dotted with oil from me applying carelessly or kicking bottles over. Keep them in your bathroom, and be careful about slipping! Contrary to belief, oil isn't impossible to get out of clothes either, so you needn't worry too much about that. Try and choose a clear oil if you're worried about yellow stains on white clothes. I must admit that I do need to bleach my sheets occasionally, as I like to cover myself in oil before bed and essentially marinate myself overnight in my white sheets.

Tips & Tricks: Oil is best absorbed into damp skin. Before you get out of the shower, apply your body oil to your wet skin, then pat dry with a towel and take care stepping out!

MY FAVOURITE PLANT OILS

You won't find coconut oil here, mainly because I tend to think it's a little overrated and I think we are all just a bit coconut-oiled out. It also is comedogenic and has large molecules, meaning it doesn't absorb well into your skin. I also think there are some great alternatives.

Jojoba: Technically a wax, this oil closely resembles our natural skin sebum. Jojoba oil has traditionally been used to moisturise skin and hair, stimulate hair growth and unclog blocked follicles. It's great for all skin types, including oily skin, and can be used on the scalp. Jojoba regulates skin oil production, so it's great for people prone to breakouts.

Rosehip: Rosehip oil has a pinky-orange colour because of its high concentration of vitamin A–containing carotenoids (which are great for the long-term health of your skin). When rosehip oil is processed, it loses its colour and, in turn, many of its benefits. Generally, the richer and darker the colour the oil is, the more skin-loving antioxidants it has. Rosehip oil is also packed with vitamin C, along with super-nourishing omega 3, 6, 7 and 9 fatty acids.

Hemp seed: You can recognise hemp seed oil by its strong, earthy smell and deep green colour. This recently popular oil is known for its anti-inflammatory benefits. It's not to be confused with hemp oil, which includes cannabidiol (CBD) oil. Hemp seed oil is also high in omega 3, 6 and 9 fatty acids. Because it's so good at helping with inflammation, this is a great one to combine with vitamin A or retinol products (page 53), which can be irritating.

Sweet almond: This is chock-a-block full of vitamins D and E, as well as magnesium and calcium. Sweet almond oil is inexpensive and has a golden colour and nutty aroma. This is a great oil for massage, but if you're sensitive to nuts, you'll want to steer clear of this one. Sweet almond oil has also been used for rashes and spider vein reduction.

Stick with sweet almond oil and avoid using bitter almond oil, which is made for its scent and flavour properties, not for its skin benefits. The sweet variety is a carrier oil used for cosmetic purposes, because the bitter variety produces a harmful component when processed. Although sweet almond oil is beneficial, if it's the first or second most used ingredient in an expensive skincare product, then it may be there as a filler, meaning the product's value for money isn't great.

Olive: For good reason, this oil was referred to as liquid gold by the Greek poet Homer. Cutting down olive trees was even punishable by death during the 6th century. Beware of impostors when it comes to olive oil – quality really does matter, and there are lots of oils that say they are olive when they are actually a mixture of other oils.

A few years ago I went on a holiday to Italy with a group of people, I forgot to bring my body moisturiser, and there was no way I was going to use the minuscule amount of face moisturiser I had on my body. Olive oil to the rescue! I was the weirdo who would go up to the kitchen every morning to moisturise. I will never forget when a friend of mine walked into the room and saw me decanting a big bottle of olive oil into my hand …

Olive oil is a great all-round skin oil. A great-quality and least-processed extra-virgin oil will have a deep green colour and robust, delicious scent. Olive oil is known for being a wrinkle remedy, and is used to produce a vegan squalane (known for its moisturising properties) that is beautiful on your skin. It also makes your skin feel deliciously smooth.

....

Tips & Tricks: Olive oil is heat sensitive and turns into a toxic trans fat when we cook with it. You're much better off using ghee or coconut oil if you're frying food!

Chai spice body oil

For: Skin and hair in need of some amazing-smelling, moisturising love.

½ cup sweet almond oil
½ cup grapeseed oil
2 vanilla beans
⅓ cup chai mix

Option: Make your own chai mix! There's no need to grind the following spices, just add them whole in the recipe:
¼ cup black tea leaves
1 tablespoon green
  cardamom pods
1 teaspoon whole cloves
2 cinnamon sticks
1 whole star anise

Chai is my favourite hot drink, especially since I don't drink coffee. The spicy cinnamon flavour brings back memories, like wandering through the flea markets in London on a cold autumn day. Alas, I don't travel like I used to … but the smell of chai brings me right back. There's something about the combination of spices that make up a chai that's soothing, comforting and totally delicious.

Sweet almond oil gives you a vitamin E boost and black tea is rich in vitamin C. Cloves have the highest antioxidant content of any spice or herb in the world. Infuse them into teas or body oils whenever you can. This recipe requires double boiling, which I generally try to avoid, purely because it's a little bit more fiddly. However, it's necessary here with the delicate nature of the spices and the gentle oil infusion process.

To make: Find a heatproof bowl that fits on top of one of your saucepans. Pour the almond oil and grapeseed oil into the bowl.

Pour a few centimetres of water into the saucepan – enough so that the bowl only touches the water slightly when placed on top of the saucepan. Warm the water until it boils, then reduce to a low heat.

Place the oil-filled bowl on top of the saucepan, keeping the heat on low.

Scrape the seeds from the vanilla beans and add them to the oil. Add the chai mix and stir occasionally. Keep on a low heat and let the spices infuse for 10–20 minutes.

Remove the bowl from the saucepan and strain the oil, discarding the spices. Pour the oil into a glass container and allow to cool.

To use: Easy! Apply like any other body oil. If you're using it in your hair, apply it to damp or dry hair and leave it in for 20 minutes before washing out.

You can use this oil as often as you like. It's got a nice wintery vibe, so it's certainly one for the colder months.

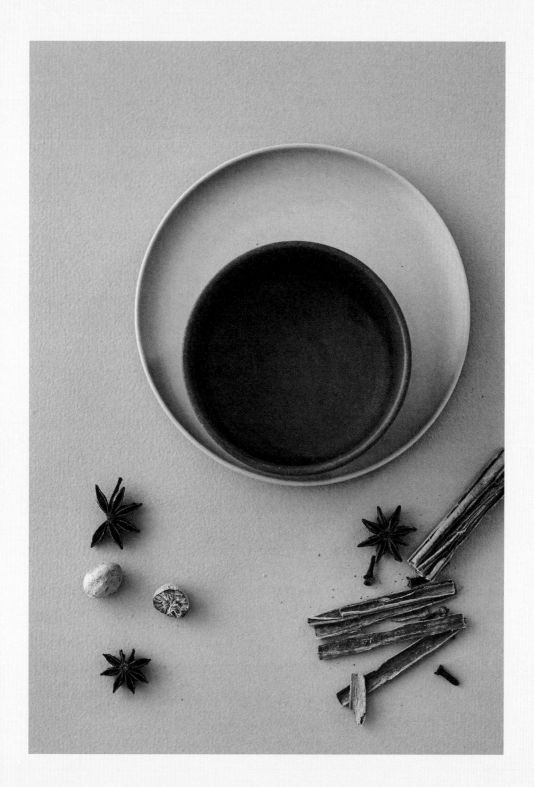

Shimmery body oil

For: A nourishing body oil with a beautiful shimmer for all skin types.

I've always loved anything with a bit of sparkle. Why use a standard body oil when you can add some shimmer? This recipe isn't too oily on the skin, it sinks in. With its shimmery glow, it is a beautiful one for summer. You can use it all over your body, but it's especially beautiful on your shoulders and legs. If you want it to have an extra summery note, then add a couple of drops of jasmine essential oil. Mica powder, which you can find online, is a mineral-based shimmer and safe to use all over your body.

1 vanilla bean
½ cup sweet almond oil
¼ cup jojoba oil
2 teaspoons silver, gold or bronze mica powder

To make: Scrape the vanilla seeds from the bean into a bowl and add the remaining ingredients.

Stir until combined, then pour the mixture into a mist spray bottle or pump bottle.

To use: Apply like a body oil, paying special attention to your shoulders, collarbone and legs. Be careful if you're wearing white or light colours – the bronze- and gold-coloured mica can stain. You can add more or less mica powder if you want to enhance or decrease the shimmer.

Use whenever you want an extra glow.

Essential oils

I am cautious to talk about essential oils here as I feel it could end up being half the book, so I'll keep it short and sweet.

Essential oils are used to enhance physical and emotional health, and they are damn fun to play with. Have you ever found that some smells can take you back to certain times in your life? That's because scents make their way to the limbic system in our brains, which is associated with memory and emotion.

1. **Frankincense:** This one gives off holy vibes, probably because it's referenced in the Bible as a gift brought to baby Jesus. The scent does have church connotations, but, overall, it gives you a sense of strength, resilience and wellbeing. I have a friend who loves how frankincense lifts her mood – she puts a drop on the soles of her feet every day.

2. **Lemon myrtle:** When I was nineteen and left home to travel for a couple of years, I brought along a bottle of lemon myrtle essential oil. It reminds me of Australia, and the smell is instantly comforting to me.

3. **Geranium:** This wonder oil can be used for your beauty in so many ways. It's great for skin and has a beautiful, feminine floral scent. I wear it alone as a perfume or mix it in my oil serum for my skin.

4. **Lavender:** This is a classic oil. Yes, a little of this oil helps you sleep, but don't go overboard as too much will actually end up stimulating you. It's also known to help heal burns and scars. I find lavender is like a big hug. I use it in my baths and my diffuser.

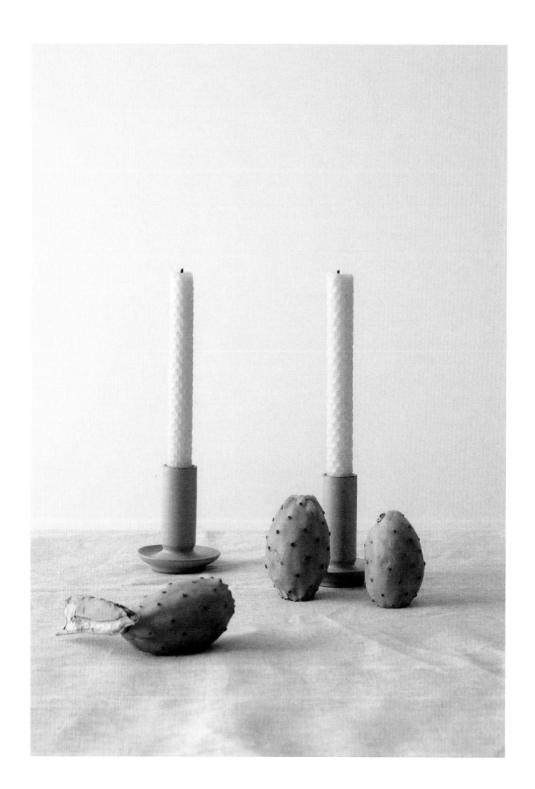

Waxes

The obvious difference between oils and waxes is that waxes are solid at room temperature. While not as versatile as plant oils, waxes can be used by themselves and are handy for making your own creations, such as the Lotion bars (page 112), because they help products keep their shape and texture.

Waxes come in two categories: plant wax and beeswax. Plant waxes include carnauba, candelilla, rice bran and sunflower wax. Carnauba wax ranges from an intense dark yellow to a light beige colour, and is available as flakes, pellets and powder. This wax is obtained from the leaves of the Brazilian carnauba palm: once dried, they are beaten to loosen the wax, then the wax is refined and bleached.

Plant waxes are highly processed; it's worth noting that extracting candelilla wax is a toxic and dangerous process that involves boiling the leaves in sulphuric acid. Because of this, beeswax is my choice of wax, even though I rarely use it. I do buy beeswax candles, because conventional scented ones are actually quite toxic – they are made from bleached or chemical-filled wax and synthetic fragrances.

Butters

Butters are really similar to waxes, but there is a slight difference in their structure. Butters are softer to the touch and melt more quickly. They don't contain water, so they can really seal in your skin's moisture.

Shea: This butter is extracted from boiled and mashed nuts from the shea tree, and is predominantly sourced from West Africa. It really had its time in the limelight a few years ago, and its popularity is largely due to its super moisturising effects and its rich vitamin A and E content.

Mango: I look forward to every mango season – I never let even the scrap of flesh around the pit escape my jaws. This butter is pressed from the dried and roasted mango pits. The husk is removed after the roasting, and then the kernels are mashed and pressed, expelling the vitamin E and antioxidant-rich butter. It feels less thick and oily than other butters or waxes. Mango butter is great for damaged or dry skin, and offers some protection against UV rays (you'll still need to use sunscreen).

Cacao: Yes – this is related to chocolate and is also known as cocoa butter. To make it, cacao beans are dried and fermented, separating the fat from the bean. If you buy raw cacao butter, you get that rich chocolate smell, although the refined version is more accessible. Rich in essential fatty acids, 70 per cent of the world's cacao butter is exported from Nigeria and Ghana. It is one of the most stable fats known, containing its own natural antioxidants. If you tend to use products slowly or live in a humid, hot environment, this butter is the choice for you.

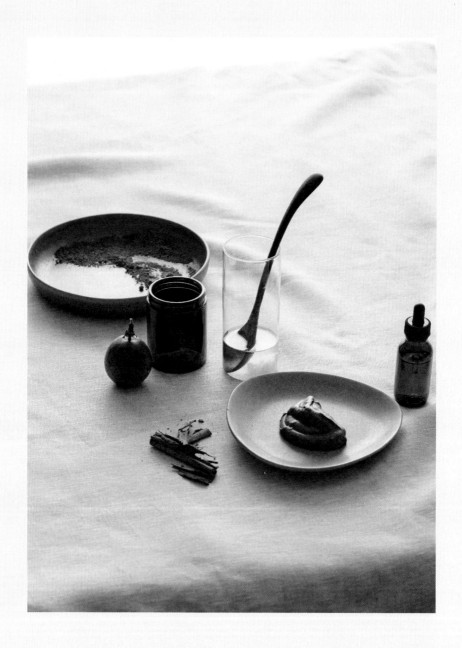

Chocolate body butter

For: Inflamed or dry skin and eczema.

If you're into chocolate like I am, the idea of rubbing it all over your body will be just fine with you. Don't worry, this body butter isn't sweet or sticky like actual chocolate, but it does have cocoa powder and cacao butter, which make it feel extra rich and nourishing. It's not as dark on the skin as it might first appear to be, but avoid wearing white or light-coloured clothes with this one.

¼ cup cacao butter
2 tablespoons shea butter
2 tablespoons extra-virgin coconut oil
2 teaspoons unsweetened organic (Dutch) cocoa powder
1 teaspoon ground cinnamon
5 drops peppermint essential oil (optional)

To make: Melt the cacao butter, shea butter and coconut oil in a saucepan over a low heat.

Remove from the heat, then stir in the cocoa powder and cinnamon. If you're using peppermint essential oil, stir it in.

Transfer to a jar and allow the mixture to cool until it becomes solid.

To use: Use as a moisturiser all over your body.

Use as often as you like (or whenever you have chocolate cravings, which in my case is about thirteen times per day).

Lotion bars

For: Skin in need of some moisturising! These bars are great to travel with.

I started making these lotion bars because I was trying to find a way to get around the travel restriction for liquids in your carry-on luggage. I also use these on my face if I'm skiing or out in rough weather. The moisturiser is nice and thick and provides an environmental barrier.

2 tablespoons beeswax pellets
2 tablespoons shea butter
1 tablespoon cold-pressed
   coconut oil
1 tablespoon avocado oil
1 tablespoon grapeseed oil
15 drops geranium essential oil
15 drops lavender essential oil
15 drops rose essential oil

To make: Melt the beeswax, shea butter and coconut oil in a saucepan over a low heat, stirring occasionally.

Once melted, turn off the heat and stir in the avocado and grapeseed oils. Add the essential oils and give it another stir.

Pour the mixture into silicone moulds. (If you don't have a silicone mould, you can use a metal cupcake tray lined with baking paper.)

Place the moulds in the fridge to set. They are best stored in the fridge too.

To use: Rub on your body. Like I said, I've used these on my face in winter too, so don't be scared of doing that if you like a thick moisturiser.

Apply as often as you like.

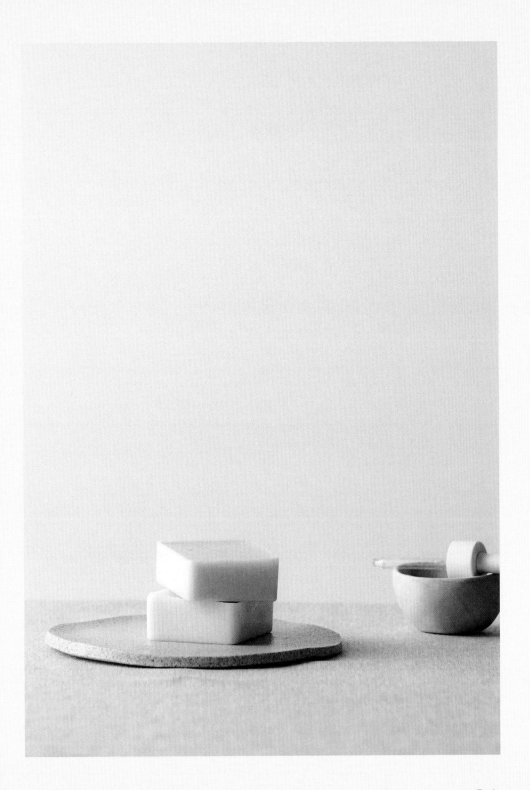

Abhyanga

When I found out about the ancient Ayurvedic oil massage technique called abhyanga, I thought it was one of the most beautiful and simple self-care practices I had ever come across. It involves only your beautiful nude body and some warm natural oil. It feels like an indulgent little treat for you to graciously give yourself.

In the West, we seem to have forgotten the importance and the power of touch. Abhyanga self-massage not only has health and beauty benefits, it is also a way to reconnect with your heavenly body. Touch has a profoundly soothing effect on our nervous system, and you only need to practise abhyanga intermittently or weekly to feel and see improvements in skin and circulation, as well as mood. I find abhyanga to be a form of meditation, with its slow ritualistic movements and the history behind the practice. I'm thinking of my friend Clara (who is an avid abhyanga lover as I write this). Her skin is beautifully healthy, and she always looks like she just got back from a tropical holiday. I think this oil massage has something to do with it.

So, how do we treat ourselves to a delicious abhyanga massage? First get the oil: if you can get your hands on some, and you can stand the smell, then black sesame oil is your number one pick – it is the traditional Ayurvedic oil used for this practice. Don't stress if you can't find it – I often use sweet almond or rosehip oil instead … it's really up to personal choice. Coconut oil is probably not a great choice: you may have to melt it first, it doesn't absorb well into the skin and is comedogenic. Warm about half a cup of

oil by placing the jar in hot water. You will also want to put some towels down. I've made the mistake of spilling body oil on my carpet many a time and have slipped on the bathroom tiles (oil on your feet and a hard floor do not mix). Use a generous amount of oil at each stage of the massage.

HOW TO PERFORM AN ABHYANGA MASSAGE

- If you want to be extra woo-woo (as I do), set intentions while you massage yourself, or show some gratitude for the organs, joints, bones and muscles of your body. After all, they work pretty hard for you with little acknowledgement.

- Start by massaging your head (you'll need to shampoo twice afterwards).

- Massage your feet as if they are the most precious tootsies in the world.

- Move up your legs, massaging upwards towards your heart. When you reach a joint, such as your knees, massage in a circular motion.

- After your legs, massage your arms. Move from your fingertips up to your shoulders, remembering to massage your elbows in a circular motion. Then massage your breasts (go on!) in a clockwise direction. You'll also want to massage your stomach this way.

- Now here's the hard part – if you can sit in the morning sun with the oil still on for 20 minutes, do that. This is hard for a few reasons: nosey neighbours getting an eyeful and winter sun being colder than it looks being the two main ones. However, it really is the icing on the cake with an abhyanga massage, so try it. Let the beautiful oil soak into your body. Yes – it feels *super* weird sitting around in the nude covered in oil – you might feel much like a piece of marinating meat. But there's something so primal and sensual about the act of touching every part of your body and then sitting still in the sun – an essential step in this sacred practice – that you'll literally feel your nervous system start to relax as if you've had a lovely glass of red wine.

- After your 20 minutes, you're ready to wash all your toxin-filled oil off. Careful stepping into the shower!

All in all, my abhyanga massages take me about an hour.

If you'd like a unique healing experience, see if there are any Ayurvedic spas you can visit. One of the great luxuries of life, in my opinion, are Ayurvedic treatments, such as shirodhara (where warm oil is poured over your forehead, specifically over your 'third eye'), abhyanga, bashpa sweda (a herb-infused steam/sauna) and garshana (Ayurvedic exfoliation and massage).

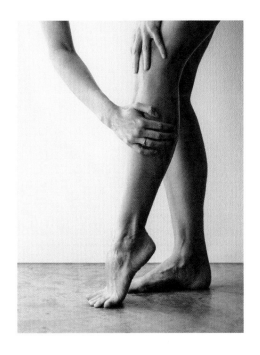

Underarms

Often forgotten, our underarms are one of the most vulnerable places on our bodies for toxins to leak in (just like they leak out!). The skin here is thinner and more sensitive, and your lymph nodes are also very close to this area. Shaving your skin makes it even easier for the nasty ingredients in conventional antiperspirants to seep in: aluminium and parabens have an express ticket to your lymph nodes, as does 'synthetic fragrance' (an ingredient that can legally hide hundreds of potentially toxic ingredients). Aluminium is a known potent neurotoxin and clogs pores.

The most effective natural deodorants, I have found, include baking soda and essential oils instead of fragrance. One thing to remember is that they are deodorants, not antiperspirants. For this reason, they won't stop you from sweating (that's what aluminium does), but they'll stop you from smelling.

Sorry to get a bit TMI – but the way you smell can be diet or hormone related. The extremely subtle pheromones released in sweat can even influence who we attract. When I met my partner, we both had a week where we were both a little 'on the nose'. It was bizarre, as neither of us are generally smelly people (I swear!). Our apocrine glands, which excrete sweat, are most active during times of excitement or nervousness, so maybe that had something to do with it.

Meat and animal fats (particularly dairy fat) have been associated with body odour, and natural chemicals in certain foods, such as cumin, onion and alcohol, are more likely to exit via the skin. So when you exercise and sweat out the damage from the night before, you're really smelling the cocktails you drank! BO can also mean an overgrowth of candida in your digestive tract. You can treat this with diet changes and supplements, but colonics are also useful. A word of warning – they aren't for the faint-hearted.

A traditional remedy for body odour is to wipe your underarms at bedtime with a cloth saturated in lemon juice. It's thought that the juice balances your pH, inactivating the bacteria responsible for the pong. Along with your natural deodorant in the morning and some essential oils for perfume, you'll be feeling (and smelling) like a goddess.

To treat body odour, you really need a holistic approach where you look at what's going on emotionally and physically. If you think anxiety could be behind your BO, supplements of magnesium, valerian or passionflower can help. Chlorophyll (which can be found as a green powder) is also known to deodorise from within.

....

Tips & Tricks: A calendula nappy rash cream can soothe a shaving rash, but this usually disappears on its own. If it doesn't, it could be something a little nastier like dermatitis. Either way, avoid conventional antiperspirants.

Deodorant

For: Preventing body odour.

¼ cup bicarbonate of soda
(baking soda)

¼ cup arrowroot powder

2 tablespoons melted virgin
coconut oil

2 tablespoons melted
shea butter

5 drops essential oil of
your choice (rose is
soothing; sandalwood
provides a beautiful
androgynous scent)

I'm only including one deodorant recipe, because I find that you need to try a few from a health store to figure out what ingredients work best for you. Generally, you'll be looking to avoid anything with aluminium or 'fragrance'. Don't forget, natural deodorants generally are not antiperspirants; they stop you from smelling but do not block your sweat glands.

To make: Combine all the ingredients together in a bowl. Keep in an airtight container.

To use: Apply a thin layer to your armpits.

Use daily.

Rose and jasmine body mist

For: A light fragrance or
a cooling mist in summer.

1 small handful of fresh
jasmine flowers

1 cup water

3 tablespoons rosewater
or rose hydrosol

10 drops rose or geranium
essential oil

3 drops vanilla planifolia oil

Perfumes are full of toxic ingredients, so I always recommend using essential oils where possible. Of course, you can mix up all different essential oils, but this rose and jasmine combination is a sweet, simple one to start with.

To make: Gently rinse the jasmine flowers, being careful not to bruise them. In a container that has a lid, combine the flowers and the water, cover the container and let the water infuse overnight at room temperature.

Remove the flowers from the water. Combine ½ cup of the jasmine-infused water with the remaining ingredients in a mist spray bottle.

Pour the remaining jasmine water into another mist spray bottle for when you need a pick-me-up.

To use: Mist on your body or clothes.

Use as often as you like.

Floral fairy dust

For: Use as a body powder, baby powder or even as a dry shampoo!

¼ cup dried rose petals
¼ cup dried jasmine flowers
¼ cup dried lavender flowers
1 cup arrowroot powder
1 teaspoon mica powder
  (optional – if you like
  shimmer)

I love using this powder. It makes me feel feminine and gives me goddess vibes. I always find flowers to be an instant mood lifter, so the more I have in my life, the better.

To make: Blitz the flowers in a blender or coffee grinder to form a fine powder.

Add the arrowroot powder (and mica powder if you're using it) and stir to combine.

Keep in a re-purposed herb shaker or old face powder container.

To use: If you are using a herb shaker, you can just turn it upside down and gently let some out. If you can only find a regular container, that's OK. Just make sure it's airtight and apply the powder with a make-up brush.

Use daily.

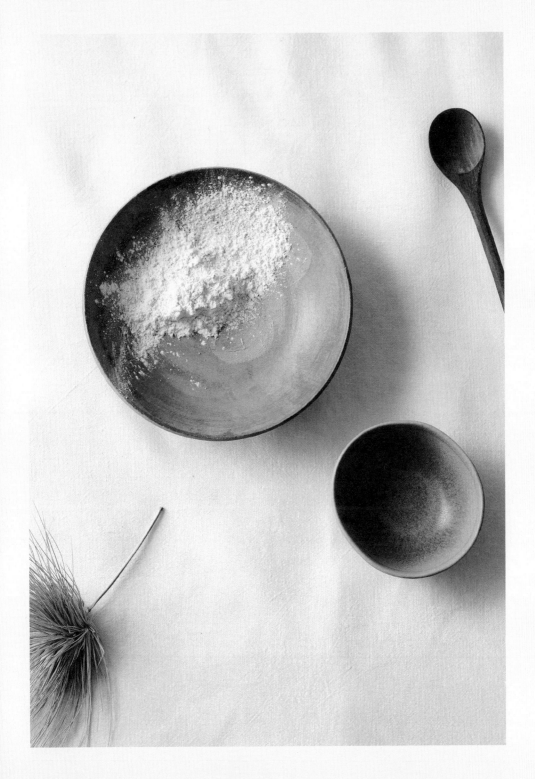

Sun care

Sunscreen must be one of the most misunderstood topics in beauty. There are some simple sunscreen facts that, in my opinion, are essential to know. If there is one thing you don't want to get wrong, it's sun protection. One of the things that really moved me towards using a mineral sunscreen was learning about all the toxic sun blockers and how they work. The chemical sun-blocking ingredients you find in conventional sunscreens (the ones you're most likely to find on the shelves) are known to be allergens, oestrogen mimickers and endocrine disruptors. A common ingredient, oxybenzone, has been shown to be cancer-causing, but only when exposed to sunlight!

These ingredients are really not advisable for use, because even tiny doses can interfere with our bodies. Most conventional sunscreens are absorbed by the skin, meaning that the product can also pass into the bloodstream. Among the mysterious blend of ingredients in a conventional sunscreen, you're sure to find some chemical-based preservatives and fragrance, such as that fake coconut scent you may love so much. Yummy – not!

Another case for avoiding conventional sunscreens is that the ingredients have been shown to contribute to the death of coral reefs. Oxybenzone and octinoxate accelerate coral bleaching; Hawaii passed a bill to ban these ingredients to protect their reefs.

Chemical sunscreens absorb sunrays, while mineral SPF formulas sit on top of skin to physically block UVA and UVB rays. Broad spectrum means a product protects against a combination of UVA rays, which contribute to skin ageing, and UVB rays, which cause sunburn.

Proper application is just as important as, if not more than, SPF level. Adequate coverage and frequent reapplying is really where it's at. Contrary to popular belief, SPF amounts are not linear. SPF 30 is *not* double the protection of SPF 15. A SPF 30 sunscreen, when applied properly, can give better protection than a SPF 50+ sunscreen that is applied too thinly or not frequently enough. It'll also expose you to lower levels of toxic sun-blocking ingredients.

I stick to a natural BB cream with SPF 30 for my face during the day (layered over my vitamin C serum and moisturiser). I keep a SPF 30 bottle in my car and put it on the back of my hands before driving. For my body, I also use SPF 30+, and reapply frequently.

....

Tips & Tricks: When you apply sunscreen, don't forget about your décolletage, neck and ears. Also, as my first-grade teacher taught me, the back of your hands are just as important as your face.

Mineral sun-blocking ingredients, such as titanium dioxide and zinc oxide, are generally much safer than the ingredients in chemical sunscreens, although it's still recommended that you don't use them in a fine mist spray bottle as the particles can make you sick if inhaled. Some can leave a white cast, but newer mineral sunscreens are significantly improved, and you can find tinted versions too. You can also buy zinc sticks that are small enough to keep in your purse. In addition to being safer, zinc oxide is also a soothing skin ingredient. I always used to get a rash about five days into wearing a conventional sunscreen; I have never had this problem using a mineral sunscreen.

A friend of mine recently got badly sunburnt while on a run on their farm. The usual go-to treatment for sunburn is, of course, aloe vera. You can only imagine the look on my face when my friend showed me the brand-name moisturiser – with aloe vera scent – they were using to soothe the burn. This product contained approximately 0.05 per cent aloe vera in a thick lotion – the worst thing for sunburn as it traps the heat. You are best to find a genuine plant extract of aloe vera gel with no other ingredients. Health food stores and some pharmacies usually stock this or just get it from the plant itself. Another trick is mixing a paste with some apple-cider vinegar and baking soda and adding it to the burn as a mask for a few minutes.

....

Tips & Tricks: Glass filters UVB but allows UVA to flow through; you're not protected from the ageing sunrays through your office or car windows.

The case for sun exposure

Everything on this earth exists thanks to the sun. Sometimes our fear of the big ball of flames above us overshadows the appreciation we should have for the star that supports and sustains all life.

We humans need a good amount of sunlight to make vitamin D for ourselves. This happens via a biochemical reaction that starts when we absorb UVB rays through our skin. Your liver and kidneys then convert the vitamin D into its active hormone, so it's also important that your liver and kidneys are in good shape.

When we aren't getting enough vitamin D, we can get bone problems, depression, hair loss and general illness. The excessive use of sunscreen and total avoidance of sun can mean we become deficient in vitamin D. Now, there's no doubt that too much sun can contribute to skin cancers, but I have a suspicion that the products we rub onto our skin have a bit to do with it too, particularly when they include known carcinogens. It's extremely difficult to get enough vitamin D from your diet, so building up a tolerance to sun is important. Try spending 15 minutes in the sun outside the peak UV time between 10 am and 3 pm (especially if you're sensitive to the sun) and enjoy the mood-boosting benefits of those beautiful sunrays.

If you're in the sun without sunscreen for a few minutes, I don't think there is any need to freak out. At the same time, spending half a day sunbaking isn't ideal (even with sunscreen), and it's *so* boring! Moderation is key, as with all things.

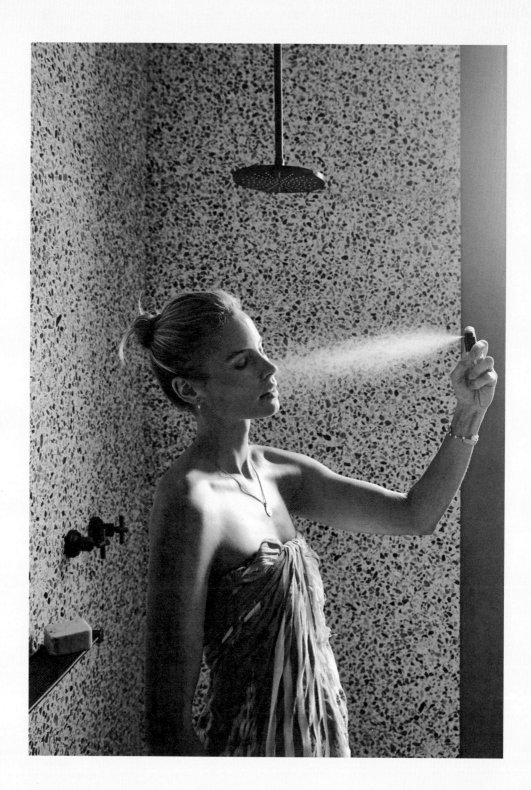

Kiwi scrub

For: Sun-damaged skin in need of a vitamin C boost.

Scrubs are a great way to use fruit that's too old to eat. Of course, kiwifruit has health benefits we can reap when we eat it, but we can also enjoy some of those benefits when using it topically. The vitamin C and E content in kiwifruit make it a useful scrub ingredient. The oats are nourishing and soothing for your skin, and frankincense is known for its rejuvenating properties.

⅓ cup Himalayan pink salt
⅓ cup rolled (porridge) oats
¼ cup sweet almond oil
1 kiwifruit, peeled and mashed
1–2 drops frankincense
   essential oil

To make: Combine all the ingredients in a bowl and mix thoroughly.

To use: Rub in a circular motion before your shower or in the shower (avoid being directly under the water).

Use three times a week.

Too-much-sun rescue spray

For: A lobster-red sunburn.

We've all been there. And if you're like me, then you'll have been there way too many times. It's looking in the mirror after a day at the beach and wondering if your skin will ever be the same again, or maybe you wake up the next day looking 40 years older. 'It'll turn into a tan,' they will say, but everybody knows you're about to shed a year's worth of skin in a week. Now, I'm talking about a bad sunburn here, but burns don't have to be that bad to be extremely painful. This spray will help decrease the pain immediately as well as heal the skin. Don't forget mineral sunscreen next time!

¼ cup pure aloe vera juice
   (make sure it doesn't
   have sugar, or combine
   2 tablespoons water with
   2 tablespoons aloe vera gel)
1 tablespoon witch hazel
1 teaspoon apple-cider vinegar
½ teaspoon vitamin E oil
8 drops lavender essential oil
5 drops peppermint essential oil

To make: Combine all the ingredients in a mist spray bottle and give it a good shake.

To use: Mist on sunburns. Don't be conservative with your use, and use it as often as you like throughout the day and night. If you're misting over your face, remember to have your eyes closed.

Use whenever you overdo it in the sun.

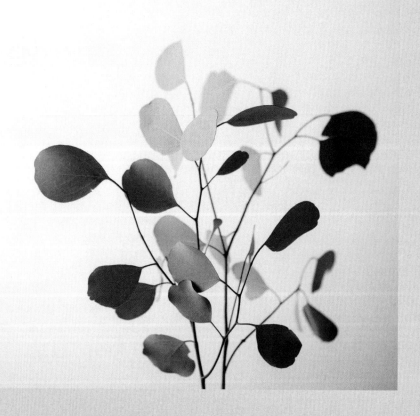

03

Hair
& Nails

You know your skin changes throughout your life, but what about your hair? Does it not deserve some of the love and attention you pay to your skin? The answer, of course, is yes. Your mane reacts really quickly to some care and loving, and there are plenty of ways that natural beauty can help. In Ayurveda, hair is seen as an extension of the powerful energy that flows up the spine, which is referred to as qi in Chinese medicine.

And how about your hands and nails? Your hands are one of the hardest working parts of your body. They're exposed to all the weathering elements and reflect our internal health just as our face does. It's important you take care of both. Even the one and only

Marie Antoinette knew that the hands were vulnerable to signs of ageing. She was known to wear gloves every night, lined with wax, almond oil and rosewater, to give her hands and nails an overnight treatment.

I'm not going to lie, I find it really hard to go 100 per cent natural on hair and nail products. I still use nail polish, although I only opt for 'cleaner' versions. As for haircare – there is some exciting progress here, with newer brands proving they can be just as effective without the toxins. It's not about being super strict and deciding to throw away all your hair and nail products, but making a couple of changes where you can.

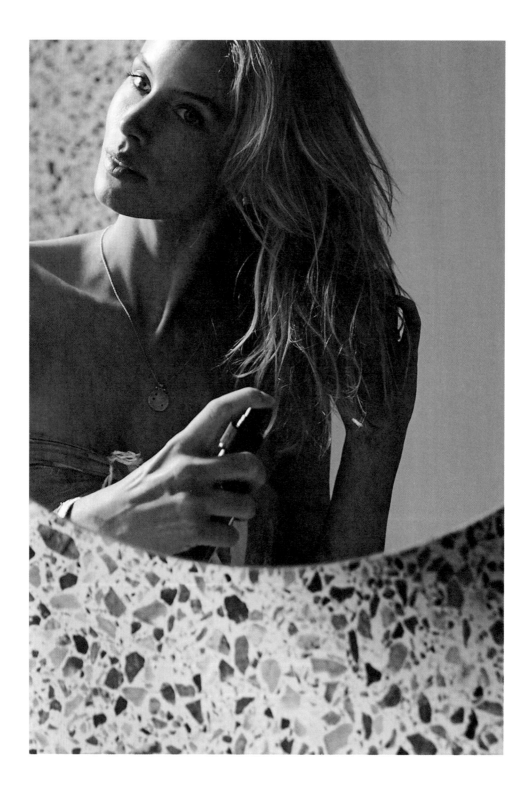

The Botanical Beauty Hunter

Hair

To care for the health of your hair, think beyond your normal use of conditioner in the shower. Hair health isn't about just beautifying the long strands of hair but also about nourishing the follicles at the roots that hold your hair in place.

More than a decade of modelling and under-eating absolutely wrecked my hair. I wasn't getting the nutrients I needed, and my hair was being hot-ironed or backcombed every day. After a regime that included regular natural hair oil treatments, supplements and a healthier diet, my hair is now unrecognisable. My friends comment on how much thicker and healthier it is, and it grows way faster than the hair of anyone else I know!

Natural haircare can be a tricky topic to navigate through. To be honest, I've found it hard to switch to completely natural haircare (I just *cannot* let go of my volumising spray). However, the best thing about making your own haircare products is that the benefits are so great (and instant), and you can use them alongside your normal shampoo and conditioner if you find natural haircare doesn't work for you just yet.

Tips & Tricks: Since I was a child, my mum's insisted I sleep on a satin or silk pillowcase, because my fine hair used to get extremely matted. I remember my poor mum spending hours with a bottle of detangling spray trying to get the knots and Blu Tack out (I had a habit of storing this in my hair!). Nowadays, they say silk pillowcases help prevent wrinkles. This sounds pretty far-fetched to me, but they feel great to sleep on nonetheless!

There are some ingredients in haircare that you really must try to avoid. Propylene glycol is used as a solvent, but it's also the active component in antifreeze. Sulfates are detergents that strip your body and hair of all their natural oils when added to personal care products. They are known to be irritating and over-clean your hair, causing it to become brittle. Try to steer clear of parabens and fragrance too, although I know it's hard when it comes to haircare. The toxic ingredients in hair products can feel like they are helping, but they really strip natural oils from the hair and scalp, leaving both seriously dry. On the other hand, moisturising hair products can leave behind a heavy, waxy build-up on both your hair and scalp, slowing hair growth.

Healthy hair food

Good-quality nutrition provides us with the bulk of what we need. In saying this, we now have the ability to be clearer than ever on what nutrients we are lacking, thanks to the plethora of testing methods available. Supplements do make a difference. In terms of my skin and hair, I can put my hand on my heart and say that I've noticed a huge difference when I have supplemented my diet, but that came with changes in what I was eating too. If you aren't well nourished, your hair won't be either. So, make sure you're eating enough good-quality healthy fats and protein. There are a couple of winning nutrients you'll want to increase your intake of if you want healthy hair. Your hair also grows slower in winter, when the scalp is tighter, and supplements can help hair grow a little faster.

In terms of nutrition, essential fatty acids are just that – essential – for your hair. They even have been studied for their ability to reverse hair loss. Omega-3 fatty acids nourish hair at the follicles to boost strength, lustre and thickness, while soothing a dry, flaky scalp and preventing the inflammation that can result in hair loss. Chia seeds, walnuts and sardines are all healthy hair foods brimming with omega 3s.

Zinc has been known to enhance the growth of hair follicles; just get tested to make sure your body is absorbing it. Oats are rich in potassium and magnesium, promoting hair growth. If you aren't vegan and are happy to eat eggs, then they are a great source of keratin and are thought to bring lustre to your hair. Spirulina is another excellent source of keratin, so throw some of that in your smoothie.

Biotin (a.k.a. vitamin B7) stimulates keratin production, helping to build stronger hair. It's thought biotin can slow the greying of hair and baldness, and even improve eczema. Biotin is available in supplement form and is also found plentifully in whole-grain rice, cabbage, egg yolks and onion.

Silica is one of the more known minerals for natural beauty health, revered for its ability to build up collagen in the body and speed up hair and nail growth. It's what holds crystals, rocks and sand together. It also makes up diatomaceous earth, a great ingredient for use in clay masks. I've dabbled in taking silica gel as a short-term treatment, which did help, although the look and taste of this suspect paste was not great. Eating brown rice is a better option for silica than drinking it in supplement form However, silica infused with horsetail (don't freak out, it's just a herb) is the superior choice if you can find it.

Hair treatments

It's certainly not hard to diagnose dry hair. Brittle strands and split ends that break easily are often accompanied by an inflamed scalp. Try not to wash your hair too much if it's already dry. I know it can get a bit yuck, but it's good to let the natural oils build up for a couple of days. Just throw your hair in a slicked-back ponytail and nobody will bat an eyelid. Use oil treatments like castor, borage, sunflower and jojoba, and make sure you're getting enough omega-3 fatty acids in your diet! The most helpful essential oils for dry hair include geranium and sandalwood, but use them diluted in a plant oil like the ones mentioned on pages 102–103.

Hair a bit on the oilier side? Aside from a natural dry shampoo (you can find a recipe on page 132), there are a few herbal wonders that can help. If you're blond or have fine hair, you might find you are more prone to oily hair, as you'll have more oil-producing glands. It might seem counterintuitive, but putting oils on your hair can actually help if it's too oily. Hazelnut and safflower oils mixed with small amounts of essential oils, such as bergamot, lime, sage, peppermint and thyme, can regulate your oil production. Conditioners can be heavy on your hair, particularly when they are full of silicones and filling ingredients. When you condition your hair, focus only on the strands and avoid the roots to not weigh your hair down. Zinc supplements as well as vitamin A and C supplements can also help balance your oil production. If you haven't tried a herbal hair rinse (page 132) on oily hair, I would advise you try it. It cleans both your scalp and your hair strands.

Camellia oil is reputed to have been used by geishas for centuries, to ensure their hair stayed silky soft and shiny. Traditionally called tsubaki oil, it is rich in fatty acids, such as omega 6 and omega 9, that make it beautifully nourishing for both hair and skin. Traditionally, the oil is applied to damp hair, either by hand or with a special Japanese wood comb.

Shiro abhyanga is a traditional Ayurvedic scalp massage technique that helps stimulate circulation and is thought to promote a restful sleep and help dissolve stress (one of the leading causes of hair loss). You can perform this scalp massage at home by simply massaging some warm oil (preferably black sesame, but any plant oil will work) into your scalp in a clockwise motion with your nails. It's going to feel about a billion times better when someone else does it for you, so try to persuade someone into doing it! Leave the oil in for 20 minutes and then just wash it out.

Tips & Tricks: Been swimming in a chlorine pool? You can neutralise chlorine by spraying your hair with a mixture of ½ teaspoon vitamin C powder dissolved in ½ cup of water.

3 key topical botanicals for hair health

1. **Castor oil:** The hair health super oil. This oil treatment has worked far better than any supplement I have taken for my hair. You can buy it as part of a blend or as a standalone ingredient. Massage it into your scalp and hair and sleep with it in overnight.

2. **Rosemary:** Whether it's in essential oil form or as a rinse (it goes great with apple-cider vinegar!), rosemary looks after your hair and scalp by reducing scalp inflammation and dandruff.

3. **Honey:** It's an odd feeling pouring honey into your hair (it's best to heat it slightly first), but its humectant properties mean it can help lock moisture into your strands before being rinsed out.

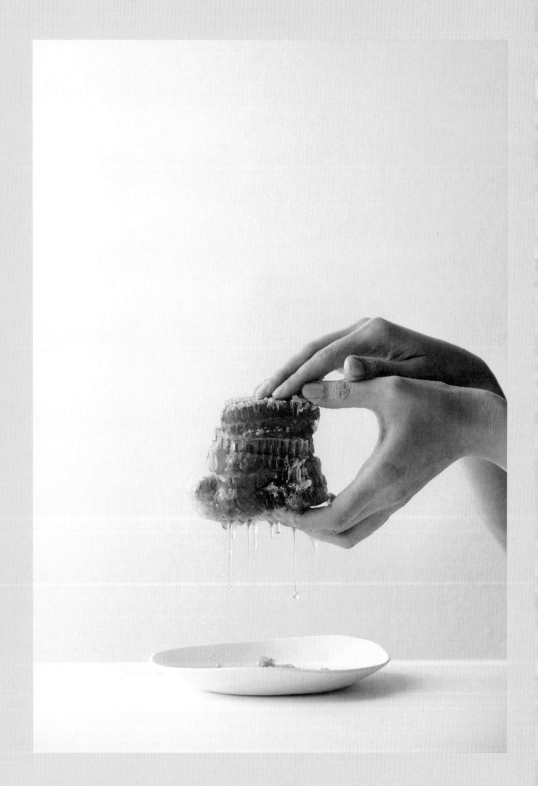

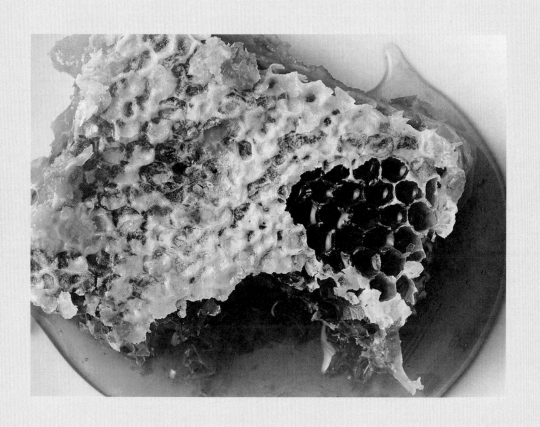

Herbal hair rinse

For: A nourishing herbal boost – like a wheatgrass shot for your hair.

If you don't have time for a hair oil treatment, then a herbal hair rinse may be for you. You'll still get the benefits of the herbs on your hair and scalp, without the time or mess that a hair oil can bring, because there's no need to shampoo after using it.

Apple-cider vinegar has been used for centuries to bring a healthy shine and lustre to your hair, and rosemary has been known to do a similar thing, while also benefiting your scalp.

2 cups water
¼ cup dried rosemary
¼ cup dried lavender
¼ cup dried basil
¼ cup apple-cider vinegar

To make: Bring the water to the boil in a saucepan and add the herbs.

Remove from the heat immediately, add the apple-cider vinegar, and let the herbs infuse for 90 minutes before straining.

To use: Pour the entire rinse on your hair in the shower after you have conditioned it, then rinse it off after 2 minutes.

Use once or twice a week.

Dry shampoo for blond and brown hair

For: Hair that you don't have time to wash! This powder also gives a slight volume boost.

Dry shampoo is great not just because it keeps your hair looking good in between washes – it's also my secret weapon for touching up regrowth. You can tailor the scent and even the colour for your hair by making it yourself.

1 tablespoon cornstarch powder
1 tablespoon arrowroot powder
3 drops essential oil (lavender and geranium both work well, but it's totally up to you)

Option for dark hair: Add 1 tablespoon unsweetened (Dutch) cocoa powder; adjust the amount to match your hair colour.

To make: Mix all the ingredients together in a small bowl or in a herb shaker.

To use: When you apply it to the roots of your hair, you can use a powder make-up brush if you want to be super specific with covering any regrowth. Otherwise, use an old herb shaker and comb through your hair after applying it.

Use whenever you have oily hair that you can't be bothered washing.

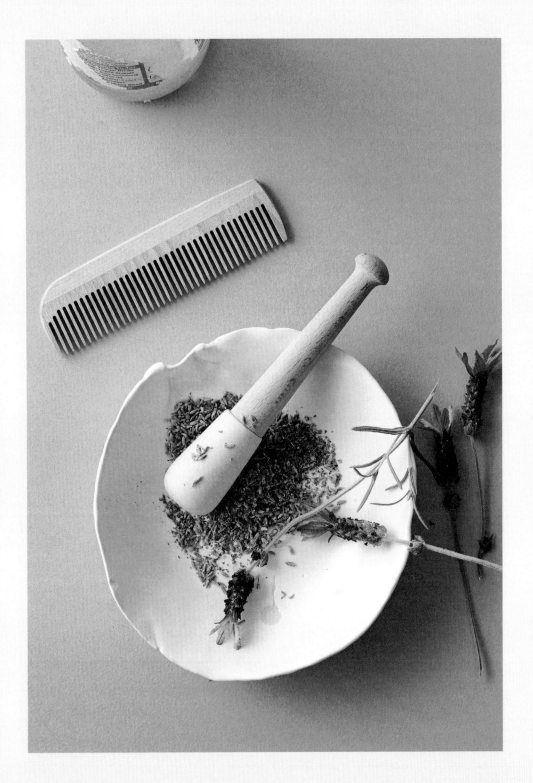

Coconut oil and beeswax hair gel

For: A natural alternative to sprays and gels.

3 tablespoons beeswax pellets
3 tablespoons coconut oil
1 tablespoon castor oil
10–20 drops of essential oils
  of your choice

The perfect slicked-back ponytail is not easy to achieve. Between the flyaways and baby hairs, it can be a pretty frustrating style to accomplish. Enter this hair gel with coconut oil and beeswax. You'll get the treatment benefits of the beeswax, coconut oil and the essential oils, which are also known for their hair benefits.

To make: Melt the beeswax and coconut oil in a double boiler (see page 104 for the method) or in a saucepan over a very low heat.

Remove from the heat and let it cool for about 5 minutes. Add the castor oil and essential oils of your choosing and stir. Pour into a jar.

To use: Apply to your hair and style as desired.

Use as often as you'd like.

Sea salt mist

For: A clean alternative to conventional so-called 'sea spray texture mist'.

1 tablespoon sea salt
¼ cup hot water
2 tablespoons aloe vera gel
2 tablespoons rose or
  neroli hydrosol
2–3 drops of essential
  oil of your choice

Ahhh – the always enviable beach hair. While conventional products are unnecessarily packed full of toxic ingredients, a sea salt spray made at home will give you a healthy alternative that still gives you that texturising feel.

To make: In a small bowl, dissolve the sea salt in the hot water.

Let the water cool, then add the aloe vera and floral hydrosol. Add 2–3 drops of an essential oil here too, especially if you like a stronger scent!

Pour into a spray bottle.

To use: Spritz on your hair as you blow dry. Scrunch your hair for extra volume.

Use as often as you'd like.

Ayurvedic brahmi and ginger hot oil treatment

For: Hair growth enhancement.

½ cup coconut oil
1 teaspoon brahmi powder
1 teaspoon grated ginger

The first time I had an Ayurvedic hair treatment, I had to run out with the herbal oil still on my scalp to catch a flight. The oil was super strong smelling, and I must admit I did get a few funny looks at the airport. Since then, I have found it much more convenient to try Ayurvedic hair treatments in the comfort of my own home.

If you can get your hands on some beautiful medicated oils from an Ayurvedic practitioner then that is ideal, but this DIY hair oil will give you a taste of Ayurveda without having to visit a clinic.

Brahmi has antioxidant properties, known to reduce hair loss and promote growth and strength in your hair. The ginger stimulates and revitalises the scalp.

To make: Melt the coconut oil in a double boiler (see page 104 for the method) or a saucepan over a very low heat. Add the brahmi powder and grated ginger. Stir for a few seconds until combined, then remove the mixture from the heat.

To use: Massage into your scalp and hair while it's still warm. Leave in for 20 minutes, then wash out with shampoo. Use a comb in the shower to make sure all the ginger comes out.

Use twice a month.

Scalp

When treating your hair health, it's important to go all the way to the root of your hair – your scalp. At the bottom of each hair follicle sits a bulb of cells; this is the only living part of your hair and the place where all nutrients are delivered to the rest of the hair. Vitamin E is great for your skin, but it's also great for your scalp. Seeds, nuts, greens and vegetables are all great sources of vitamin E, but it's also available in supplement form.

The dandruff that most of us experience at least mildly at some point in our lives is often just a symptom of an irritated, dry scalp. Whilst anti-dandruff shampoo will help mask the symptoms, you're better off going straight to the cause and giving your dry, flaky scalp exactly what you'd think it would need: some nourishing oil. Borage oil capsules taken three times a day after meals are thought to prevent dandruff, especially when used in conjunction with weekly hair oil treatments on your hair and scalp. A dietary supplement of biotin, zinc or evening primrose oil can also be beneficial.

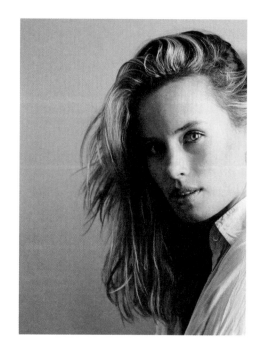

Apple–cider vinegar, tea tree and lavender dandruff cleanser

Not only will you love the natural conditioning benefits of apple-cider vinegar, but its cleansing and antibacterial properties will help reduce dandruff. Birch leaves are soothing and tea tree oil and lemon juice further enhance the dandruff-removing properties of this hair cleanser.

For: Dandruff-prone scalps.

2 cups apple-cider vinegar
2 tablespoons birch leaves
  (you can buy this online
  in tea form)
1 tablespoon lemon juice
15 drops tea tree essential oil

To make: Bring the apple-cider vinegar to a boil in a saucepan.

Remove from the heat and add the birch leaves immediately. Let the leaves infuse for 1 hour.

Strain the vinegar, discarding the birch leaves, and add the lemon juice and tea tree essential oil. Store in a mason jar.

To use: Just add 4 tablespoons to your scalp and leave it in for 20 minutes before rinsing with water.

Use as often as you'd like.

Irritated scalp serum

Oils are heaven for an itchy or irritated scalp. We tend to forget how important the health of the scalp is for the rest of our hair. This recipe will make sure it gets the love and attention it deserves.

Rosemary is great for reducing dandruff, and lavender combats any infection. The proteins in hemp seed oil help the formation of keratin, which is essential for healthy hair.

For: Itchy or irritated scalps in need of some nourishment.

1 tablespoon hemp seed oil
1 teaspoon sesame oil
1 teaspoon jojoba oil
2 drops rosemary essential oil
2 drops lavender essential oil

To make: Combine all the ingredients in a jar – make sure you really shake them together properly.

To use: Apply to your hair and scalp and leave for 20 minutes before washing out, preferably with a sodium lauryl sulphate–free shampoo to lessen the chance of further irritation.

Use as often as you'd like.

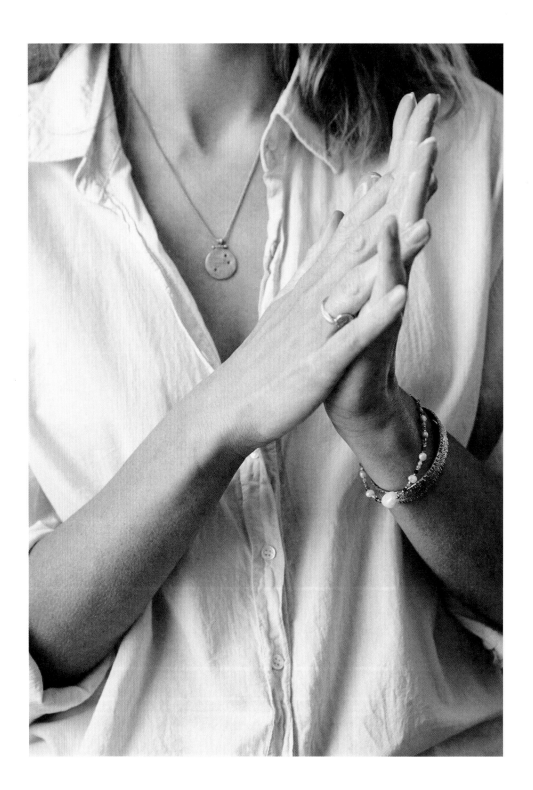

Nails

A few years ago, I saw a naturopath who asked to look at two things: my tongue and my nails. I never knew you could tell so much by a simple on-the-spot nail diagnosis. For the most part, my nails have been strong, but there have been times when they chip and become brittle, and sometimes little white specks appear and don't seem to disappear.

If you have brittle nails – and you haven't been going crazy washing dishes – you might want to look at your diet first. Iron deficiency is a common cause of brittle nails, as is vitamin A deficiency. Like our hair and skin, a less than substantial diet shows up in our nails. If you're not low in any vitamins or nutrients, it's possible (yet less likely) that you might have an underactive thyroid, in which case you'll need to go and visit your doctor. Dents in our nails can be linked to skin conditions such as psoriasis, and those white spots? If you didn't just bang your nail, consider that you may be either not absorbing zinc properly or not consuming enough of it. For more zinc, eat plenty of brazil nuts, figs and walnuts. If your nails have a slightly yellow stain, it's likely the result of too much nail polish. Give your nails a breather and gently buff them to speed up the removal of the yellow. Tea tree oil can help remedy a yellow stain.

B vitamins are crucial for nail health. You'll find that as your hair and nails are both made of keratin, so you'll experience both better hair health and nail health when you supplement one or the other. While you're onto your B vitamins, consider trying some multivitamin and mineral tablets. Minor deficiencies can be at the root of nail problems.

If chronic dry hands and cuticles are a problem, you may want to consider buying some cotton gloves you can sleep in. You can make a beautiful nourishing butter (recipe on page 142) for your hands and sleep with the gloves on overnight. The last time I was in the US, I bought some disposable gloves and socks, and I'm not going to lie – it felt totally bizarre to sleep in them, but my hands and feet were soft as a baby's bottom the next day.

....

Top 5 foods for nails

1. Leafy green vegetables
2. Spinach
3. Apricots
4. Oily fish
5. Nuts and seeds

....

Tips & Tricks: What are you using for cleaning? Harsh products can damage our health in more ways than one. They are not safe to inhale and can wreak havoc on our skin and ruin our nails. Try to switch to natural cleaning products!

The truth about nail polish

Think there's no harm in nail polish? Your nails are hard and therefore don't absorb? I can see your logic, but unfortunately, it's not true; your nails are porous and absorb what you put onto them.

Nail polish is much like natural haircare – I find switching to completely natural really difficult with both. There are no 100 per cent natural nail polishes, but there are newer, less toxic options.

Most nail polishes contain a number of chemicals. A film-former, usually cellulose acetate butyrate, makes the product hard and shiny when it dries. To make this film tough, a secondary film-former, such as formaldehyde resin (a proven carcinogen), is used. To prevent chips and cracks, one or more plasticisers, including dibutyl phthalate, may be included. Solvents like butyl acetate and toluene are used to help products glide on more smoothly.

Formaldehyde can be absorbed through the skin and nail beds, but it's triple trouble when you're in a nail salon, as it can also be inhaled. (I watched a documentary recently that showed the lack of regulation for manicure and pedicure specialists, who work all day long practically bathing themselves in a cloud of toxic ingredients without sufficient protection, such as face masks.) Formaldehyde has been linked to leukaemia and severe allergic reactions, hence it's used very rarely in the European Union, where there are stricter regulations on the use of chemicals in cosmetics.

Phthalates help the nail polish stay smooth on application, but if given the choice, I'd certainly choose lumpy nail polish over phthalates! A 2007 study by pathologists found that women exposed to phthalates when pregnant have increased incidence of boys born with missing testes (a.k.a. cryptorchidism). Other researchers in Denmark have found that breast milk can be contaminated with phthalates, directly influencing the hormone levels of newborn boys. It goes without saying, if you're thinking about having a baby or you're pregnant, getting your nails done will just have to be put on hold. A clean hand without nail polish is, in my opinion, more beautiful than a thick layer of fake lacquer anyway.

After reading the above, you're probably wanting to remove your nail polish – I don't blame you. Just try and choose an acetone-free nail polish remover. Acetone is used in paint thinner and can be extremely toxic and very drying on your poor nails that are trying to emerge from being stuck under toxic lacquer for days. N-Methyl-2-pyrrolidone, found in nail polish removers, is prohibited for use in cosmetics in the European Union due to links to cancer, mutagenicity and reproductive toxicity. It's not what you want.

After all this, you might still want to use nail polish. I mean I get it – having a manicure can be an easy way to perk yourself up when you're feeling a little flat. But at the very least, do try to use a less toxic base coat. Your best option is to find a '3-free' polish, meaning they have no phthalates, toluene, or formaldehyde, none of which you would want to inhale, use on your body or otherwise come into contact with. You might have to search for them online, but they are available.

Better yet – just clean and buff the nails really well, and use a cuticle oil. I can guarantee that you will get more compliments on some healthy natural nails than you would on a manicure with three layers of polish.

The regular manicures you might be used to probably make you think you're doing the best thing to help control cuticles and help nail health, but it might be doing the opposite. The cuticle cutting can leave you susceptible to nasty infections (I've certainly had one of these before), and you might find, like me, that the less regular your manicures, the more healthy your nails. I rarely paint my nails now. I keep them in check with a regular douse of cuticle oil (which improves the health of the whole nail), as well as cutting and filing the nails as needed, and clipping cuticles when necessary. It's an easy part of your grooming routine, and I seriously don't miss sitting in nail salons waiting for my polish to dry, only to knock a nail when I get my keys out of my pocket.

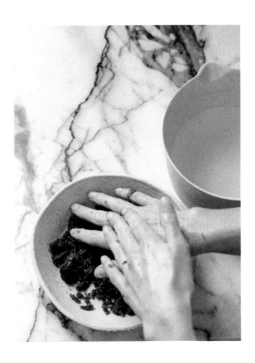

Nail-strengthening oil

For: Nails that need help!

1 tablespoon sweet almond oil
1 tablespoon olive oil
2 teaspoons vitamin E oil
5 drops lemon essential oil
5 drops frankincense
  essential oil

Regular manicures and pedicures can leave us with weak and brittle nails. Sometimes you just have to give yourself a break from the nail polish and start using some natural goodness to build the health of your nails. This oil will help bring back strength to brittle nails.

To make: Combine all the ingredients in a bowl, and store in an airtight jar.

To use: Massage the oil over your nails and cuticles and leave on for a few minutes. Wipe off any excess oil.

Use weekly.

Whisked cuticle and hand butter

For: Super dry hands and cuticles that need some extra attention.

2 tablespoons shea butter
1 tablespoon cacao butter
1 teaspoon honey
2 teaspoons rosehip oil
2 teaspoons olive oil
5 drops lavender essential oil
1 vitamin E capsule or
  about 4 drops of vitamin E oil

Cuticles and nails sometimes require a heavy-duty therapy to get them feeling their best again. This butter is just that. It's a rich treatment for both your hands and nails. Just like Marie Antoinette, you'll be leaving this on overnight if you can, so you wake up with hydrated skin in the morning.

To make: Melt the shea butter, cacao butter and honey in a saucepan over a very low heat.

Remove, let cool for 2 minutes and stir in the rosehip and olive oils. Add the lavender essential oil and break the vitamin E capsule into the mixture. Stir to combine.

Once the mixture looks as if it's almost about to start solidifying, whisk until it thickens.

To use: Apply a generous amount to your hands and put on a pair of gloves (ones that you can throw in the washing machine). Sleep with the gloves on.

Use once a week or more if desired.

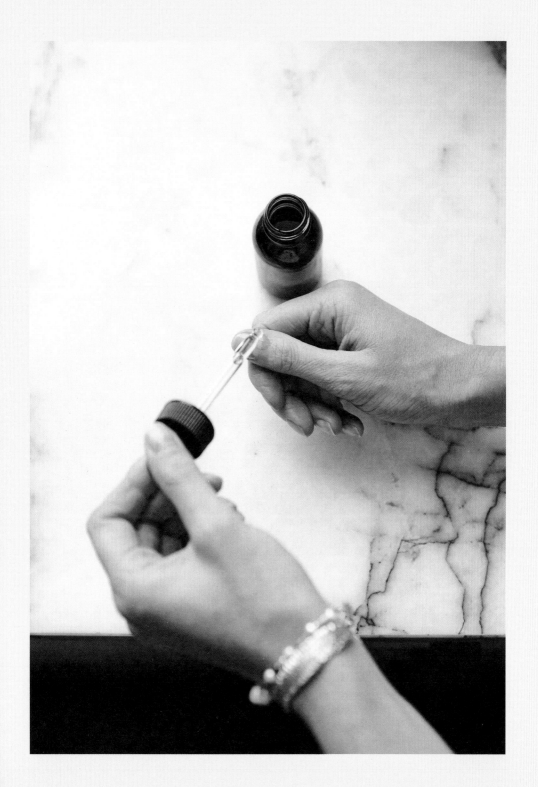

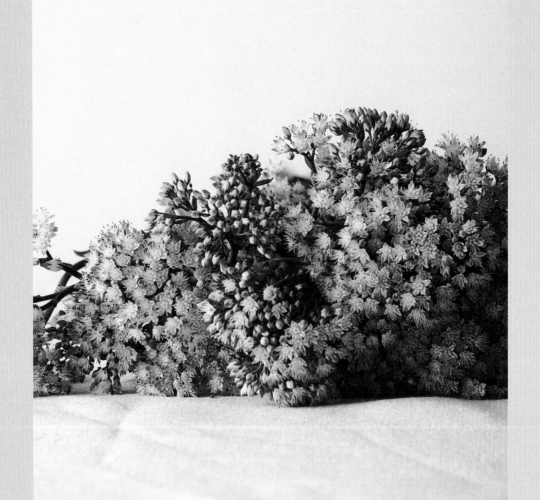

04

Self–care

I couldn't write a book about beauty and wellness that didn't talk about the topics covered in this chapter: diet and supplements, perfume and make-up, travel, and emotional wellness. This chapter will tie everything together for you so you can make some real changes to the way you look and feel, while knowing exactly which ingredients to avoid in conventional cosmetics.

Foods for your skin

Ain't no doubt about it, what we eat is reflected in how we look. For example, I went to high school with a girl who only ate pumpkin; as a result, her face and hands were literally a shade of orange. I don't think anyone would recommend eating one food group only, no matter how healthy it is. When you're eating for your health and beauty, variety is key. If you're lucky enough to have access to quality fresh produce all year round, then why not get as many nutrients as you can from the earth's bounties?

Bone broth

There are some nutrients, like vitamin B12, that you can only get from animal protein. I have a couple of long-term vegan friends who have started supplementing their diet with bone broth for health reasons. One of them was taking it to help heal major stomach issues, which it did, the other for a mineral deficiency. Protein, collagen and amino acids are all plentiful in bone broth. Since collagen is made up of eighteen amino acids, it's best to gobble up foods that provide these amino acids like bone broth does.

Tips & Tricks: Collagen-boosting amino acids can also be found plentifully in spirulina and in seafood, for example in crabs and scallops. Some people swear by taking collagen supplements, such as marine collagen peptides, although I can't say I've experienced any results myself.

Protein

Protein is like scaffolding for our skin. Our skin cell turnover decreases as we age, so it's important we continue with an adequate protein intake to help keep our skin strong.

For the non-vegans, you should know as much as you can about the animal product you're eating. Is it organic? Is it free-range? Bonus points if you know the farm it came from. 'Free-range' for chickens merely means that the animals have one square foot of space for themselves (they can still be kept in barns), so choosing a small-scale, organic family-run farm is sometimes the way to go. Some of these farms even have live cameras over their fields so you can see exactly how the animals live.

Berries

Berries are a fabulous, delicious source of vitamin C that are also low in sugar. While sugar is beneficial in scrubs and exfoliants, eating lots of sugar will not help at all in your quest for beautiful, healthy skin. Excess sugar intake encourages glycation, an irreversible natural process where sugar molecules bind to elastin and collagen, leading to premature wrinkles. It doesn't stop there, unfortunately. Sugar also causes inflammation, leading to pimples and irritation. Ever notice how you get a pimple or two in the days following a gluttonous stint? I have one right now – the result of a plethora of Christmas Day desserts.

But don't be pedantic. Eat the chocolate and drink the wine – just not too much and not too often. It's not about restricting yourself into oblivion, it's about fulfilment and satisfaction without total hedonism.

Berries are great because they are guilt-free and can be added to so many meals. I'll have some in my smoothie in the morning and then have some more after dinner. If you can buy organic, do. Berries are among the crops that are sprayed the most.

Greens

Greens, such as watercress, spinach and kale, are rich in the antioxidant plant pigments known as carotenoids, which boost immunity and protect skin cells against UV radiation. Their anti-inflammatory effects reduce the risk of heart disease and inflammation in the skin. Vitamin A helps normalise the skin's production of oil too. You can also use green superfood powders in your face masks.

Nuts

Nuts are the world's greatest snack. A word of warning – they can be hard to digest. For me, it's a fine line. If I eat a few too many nuts (macadamias are my absolute favourite), I am up for some serious bloating. Interestingly, peanuts don't seem to do the same thing, most likely because they are technically a legume. Nuts are rich in skin-loving omega-3 essential fatty acids and the amino acid called arginine, which stimulates the body to release important hormones. It's worth noting that while almonds are delicious (yes, almond milk is too), they're also unsustainable. It takes 12 litres (3 gallons) of water to produce just one almond. Yikes! Oat milk is a delicious and nutritious alternative to almond milk, as are macadamia and rice milks.

Lemons

Lemons are thought to be a liver cleanser and a vitamin C powerhouse. Vitamin C helps neutralise free radicals and helps us regenerate collagen and elastin (which bind skin cells together, giving us firm, younger-looking skin). Adding a dash of lemon to your green tea can make it easier for your body to absorb the vitamin C. Adding lemon juice on your greens will help you absorb the iron.

Lemons are one of the most alkalising foods we know of. Yes – they taste acidic, but once metabolised, the minerals they contain help alkalise and balance our body's pH levels. Most of us are way too acidic, thanks to caffeine, alcohol, poor diets and stress. Our skin will show us when our pH levels are out of whack, so trying to maintain balance with a healthy diet that includes a variety of flavours is key.

Tips & Tricks: If you have stomach or digestion problems, try chewing ½ teaspoon of fennel seeds after your meal. This ancient Indian trick helps calm your stomach.

The worth of water

I've noticed such a link between water and our beauty that I'm going to drill it into you right now. A hydrated body is your best overnight remedy for unwelcome wrinkles. When I went to boarding school in the Australian bush, we spent days hiking and carrying everything we needed in our backpacks. One of the first things we were taught was the importance of drinking more than enough water. I remember the teacher mentioning that by the time we were thirsty, our bodies had already lost 3 per cent of their water content, and by the time we had a headache, 5 per cent. Now, I don't know how true this is – but it certainly got me to drink a whole lot more! A lack of water intake can also slow our metabolism and result in the build-up of toxins in our system, which can show up on our skin. You really are gradually flushing out your system when you drink water.

And it's not just quantity; the quality of our water is also important. A friend of mine recently came up with a rash all over their torso because the water in their house was filled with heavy metals they knew nothing about. Lots of the pipes that deliver the water out of our taps are old and worn, leaching metals that can build up in our system. There are special filters that you can buy that take these metals out. There are even systems you can connect to your house so that your shower water is purified. I have a 2 litre (68 fl oz) glass jug with its own water-purifying filter. The best thing about it is that it's one of the few filters that gets rid of fluoride too.

Also, it's best to stick to stainless steel or glass bottles where you can. Ever smelled or tasted that plasticy odour from a plastic water bottle that's been left in the sun? Step away from the bottle. That's a sure sign that plastic compounds like polyethylene terephthalate are leaching into your water. Ecologically, we're all aware of the damage plastic is doing to our environment. The bottles (and all plastics) are made from petroleum as well as other carcinogens. We don't want to be consuming it or putting it on our planet.

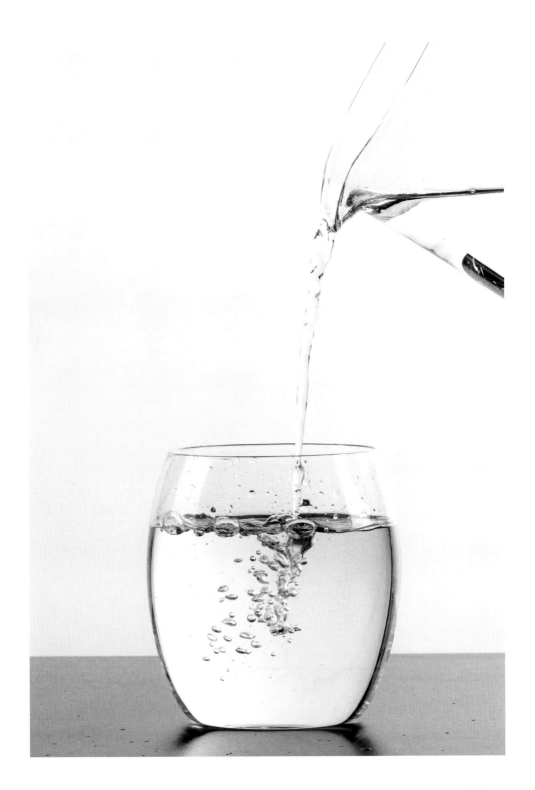

Skin–health supplements

Collagen is a protein found all through our bodies. There are many factors that determine how quickly the collagen in our skin diminishes (a standard rate is 1 per cent per year after we turn 25). Lovely holidays where we sit in the sun all day, diets where we eat too much sugar and not enough nutritious foods, and stress are all factors in how quickly collagen depletes. Fear not – it's not totally out of our control. We can manage the rate at which it depletes and keep our skin healthy with diet, skincare and in-clinic treatments such as light therapy. We can consume antioxidants to further protect our collagen from succumbing to our (wayward) lifestyles. But forget about using a skincare product with collagen in it – the molecules are too big and don't pass on into our skin at all.

I'm an avid supplement user because I have had great success with taking them to heal various health issues in the past. There are some supplements I have found beneficial no matter what my skin is going through, and these are a few that I can vouch for. None of them have to be taken as a liquid, so you don't have to worry about any foul-tasting concoctions. You might want to take them all, or just sample one or none at all. See what works for you.

Cod liver oil

Cod liver oil is the most effective and fast-acting supplement I have ever taken. I literally noticed a difference overnight in my skin, when dry skin on my neck vanished and was visibly moisturised when I woke up. If you don't have dry skin, it can still benefit you because it's thought cod liver oil can work for hyperpigmentation and boost your vitamin D level. You can drink a small amount in liquid form, but I prefer the capsules myself. I could never quite get used to the taste of fishy oil.

Cod liver oil contains omega-3 fatty acids, which help clear up inflammation, and this may be why people with acne also report that their skin clears when they start taking this supplement. But unlike fish oil, it also contains vitamin A and should be avoided if you're pregnant (or looking to be). Otherwise it's a supplement I wouldn't stop taking. You don't need to take much. I notice the difference in my skin after taking it for a day.

It's important to never consume fish oil capsules that are old, as rancid oils can actually cause inflammation. Walnuts are also full of omega-3 fatty acids, so vegans needn't miss out on the collagen-boosting benefits of omega-3 fatty acids either.

Coenzyme Q10

Coenzyme Q10 is naturally present in human skin, but once we hit 25 years of age, the production of CoQ10 declines, so this one is important to get as a supplement. CoQ10 has a variety of functions that help us look and feel our best. Conversely, low levels of CoQ10 have been associated with premature ageing. The enzyme is found in wholegrains and oily fish, and its supplement forms are relatively easy to find. If you see it in cosmetics as a topical ingredient, chances are the potency is too low to make any difference, so just stick to getting it in supplements.

Vitamin C

Vitamin C is delicious. It's also one of the only vitamins Miranda Kerr takes daily and is great for maintaining healthy tissues – not just boosting our immunity. It's almost impossible to overdose on this vitamin, which is fabulous, especially when one cup of acerola cherries contains more than 20 times the recommended daily intake for women. (The recommended daily intake for women is 75 milligrams; one cup of acerola cherries contains 1677 milligrams of vitamin C.)

If you're going to buy vitamin C supplements, it is worth buying one that is buffered and in an oil-soluble time-released Ester-C, or as L-ascorbic tablets or powder. Vitamin C is expelled from our bodies within a few hours, so these qualities help with absorption and therefore boost its effectiveness too.

....

Tips & Tricks: The dose of vitamin C to help with colds has been found to be a whopping 7000 milligrams. That's between seven to fourteen vitamin C tablets per day! If you're taking it to stop your cold, you're probably better off with a specific cold and flu tablet that has echinacea and olive leaf extract in the mix.

Zinc

Ever noticed white spots on your nails? You might be deficient in zinc. People often have trouble absorbing this skin-loving mineral that's best taken in liquid form. Not only does zinc help to look after our skin, but it also plays a large role in taking care of our immune system. Traditional sources of zinc, such as grains and meat, are just not as effective as they used to be because our modern soils are depleted of zinc and other vital minerals. Freezing vegetables causes them to lose up to 50 per cent of their zinc content too. So although you might think you're getting enough zinc from your diet, you still may need to take it as a supplement.

....

Tips & Tricks: You might notice your sense of smell and taste increase when you start taking zinc supplements. Poor tastebuds are a good sign you're low on zinc!

Body and face mapping techniques

Pimples seem to pop up everywhere, don't they? We all get them; even if you have dry skin on your face, you can still wake up with a pimple on your butt. Notice that some pimples always appear in the same place? There might be a reason. Face or body, pimples come up in certain places to tell you something, indicating deeper issues with organs. And it's not just pimples; stubborn areas with dry skin or rashes can also mean something is going on internally.

Ancient Ayurvedic and traditional Chinese medicine (TCM) both use body mapping (called mien shiang in TCM) to identify a variety of conditions. Body acne, specifically if it's on your back, chest or butt, can be attributed to hormonal changes, diet, stress and even sweat. The sebaceous glands that secrete oil (sebum) are more prominent in these places on our body, which can cause pimples to rear their ugly heads. This all makes sense, but I have found body and face mapping very helpful in working out the causes of skin conditions I experience.

Thighs

Allergies, ingrown hairs and generally sensitive skin could be to blame for acne on your thighs. It comes up as a reaction to body lotions and other bathroom products, and chemical-based laundry detergents. Folliculitis, an inflammation of the hair follicles, is also a common cause of pimples in this area. You can try experimenting with a body wash that contains chemical exfoliants (page 48), such as salicylic or glycolic acid, and switch to wearing lighter, looser pants for a little while.

Back

BACNE! We are all likely to experience some form of it at some point. It's often caused by sweat, so if you're not showering right after exercising, then you better start! Breathable clean clothes can also help. The pores on your back are more prone to clogging than pores on the face. Here, a body wash with chemical exfoliants can help. Cutting back on fried foods also helps, because diet certainly plays a part.

Butt

The dreaded butt pimple. It's not as gruesome as it sounds; it's likely just a blocked hair follicle that needs some lactic acid lovin'. It's also thought that they may be linked to digestion, so pay attention to how your stomach feels and consider some probiotics and digestive enzymes. Also don't spend too long in those yoga pants, as comfortable as they are – throw on something in a breathable cotton fabric instead.

Face mapping

As for your face, inflammation, dry skin and rashes in particular spots can be attributed to certain organs, as seen on this face diagram. If you want to discuss the skin and internal organ connection further, I would chat to a great TCM doctor or a naturopath. There's no doubt that our internal health is reflected in our skin, so it's something I would definitely be paying attention to.

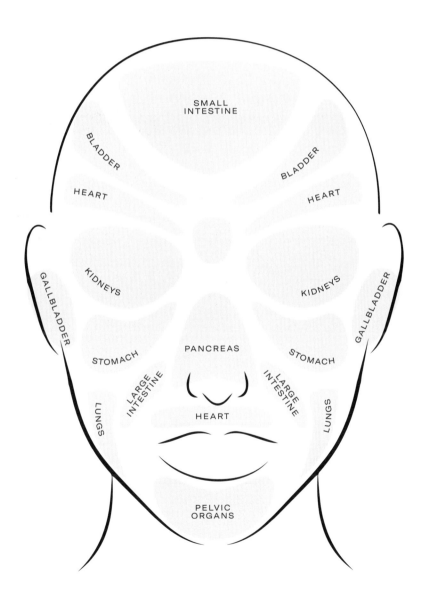

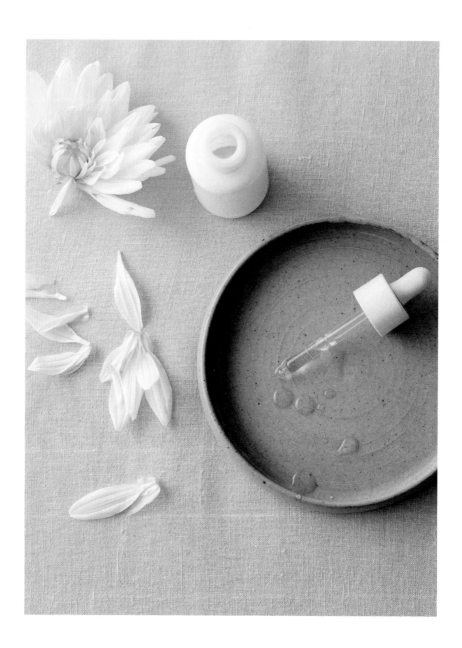

Decoding product labels

If you pay attention to the ingredient lists on the cosmetics on the shelves, you might feel like you need a chemistry degree to figure them out. That's hardly surprising if the product isn't natural, because many of the chemical names are pretty much impossible to pronounce. When the product is natural and you're still seeing long names, it may be because cosmetic companies are required to label ingredients with their scientific or INCI (International Nomenclature of Cosmetic Ingredients) names (although often, if it's a botanical ingredient, it will have its regular name on the label too).

A quick web search will tell you if an ingredient is something you want on your body or not. Ingredients on products are labelled from the most to least in terms of quantity; for example, when aqua (or water) is the first ingredient on the list, water is the main ingredient in the product. If the active or 'hero' ingredients aren't in the top quarter of the ingredient list, I'd be questioning the efficacy of the product, unless the desired ingredient is effective in very small doses (such as retinol, page 53).

There's several nasty ingredients you should avoid at all costs, and a lot of them have several names, which again might require some searching online. If you just search 'other names for lead in cosmetics', for example, you'll see what I mean.

1,4-DIOXANE (ALSO LABELLED AS SODIUM LAURETH SULFATE, PEG COMPOUNDS)

This is a cancer-causing petrochemical found in both baby and adult personal care products, and it has also been known to cause birth defects. It's found mostly in foaming products and is added to sodium lauryl ether sulfate to convert it to the less harsh laureth sulfate. It's banned for use in Canada.

GLYCOL ETHERS, LIKE ETHYLENE GLYCOL (A.K.A. PHENOXYETHANOL OR POLYETHYLENE GLYCOL)

These are used as solvents to help thin out a liquid mixture and are commonly used in certain paints. They are also found in some conventional cleaning products, brake fluid and, worryingly, cosmetics. Studies on male painters have linked exposure to certain glycol ethers to blood abnormalities and lower sperm counts.

PHTHALATES (ALSO LABELLED AS DBP, DEP AND DEHP)

There is evidence to show that phthalates are endocrine-disrupting chemicals. Again, it's the cumulative effect of these chemicals that build up from using many products over days, weeks and months that we really need to worry about. Phthalates are most commonly found in perfume, which we not only spray on our skin and clothes, but also incidentally end up inhaling. Phthalates have even been linked to early onset puberty in girls. They are banned for use in the European Union.

FRAGRANCE (ALSO LABELLED AS AROMA, PARFUM)

What a mystical term this is. It can act as a cover for companies who don't want to fully disclose their ingredients, because the term 'fragrance' can include a number of different chemicals all under the one umbrella. It's not hard to spot an immediate fragrance reaction, such as sneezing from perfume or a skin sensitivity to washing detergent. This is hardly surprising because most synthetic fragrances are derived from petroleum with scent chemicals added, as well as preservatives and solvents. There's simply no need for artificial fragrance when beautiful, beneficial essential oils exist.

PARABENS

Parabens are used as preservatives. They have reportedly been found in breast tissue and are known endocrine disruptors. They have lots of different names, including butylparaben, propylparaben, ethylparaben, methylparaben, isobutylparaben and isopropylparaben. Nowadays, there are plenty of safer ways to prevent microbial growth in cosmetics, so their use is not necessary.

OTHERS

There are multiple other ingredients to watch out for. These are just a few: phenoxyethanol, benzoyl peroxide (linked to the promotion of tumour growth), chemical UV filters (such as oxybenzone and octinoxate), hydroquinone, triclosan (a serious pesticide), lead acetate, coal tar and toluene.

Let's be honest – wouldn't it be easier to just go natural altogether and make more of your own products, thereby eliminating many of these toxic compounds from your life? You won't have the stress from worrying about what's in your beauty products, and not having to spend time decoding labels is a bonus!

....

Tips & Tricks: If you believe that nothing can be absorbed into your bloodstream through your skin, consider the effectiveness of nicotine patches for quitting smoking, or the use of oestrogen patches in hormone replacement therapy. Our skin is super absorbent and our largest organ!

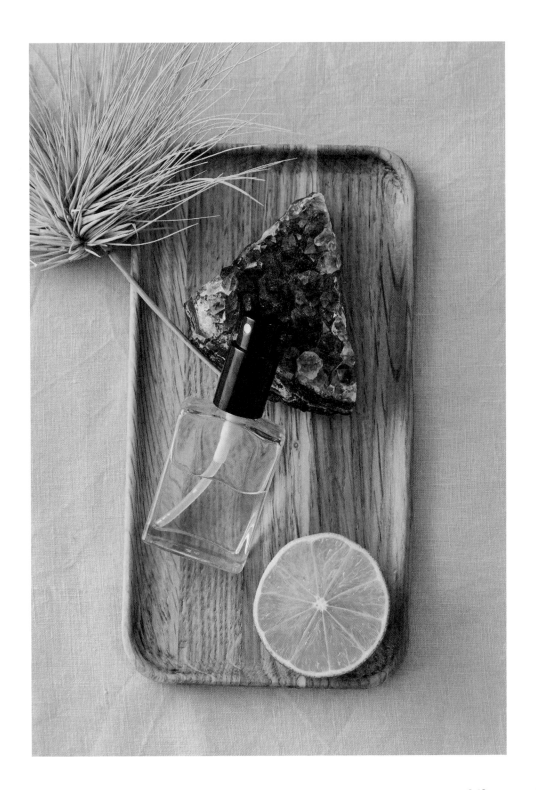

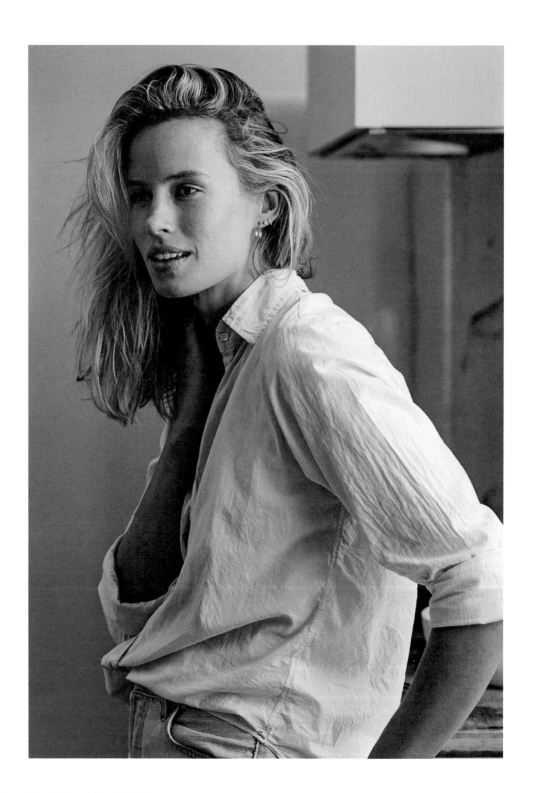

The Botanical Beauty Hunter

Going natural with perfume and make-up

Persian doctor Avicenna (AD 980–1037) is thought to be one of the first to extract fragrance – he manufactured rosewater and musk. The Romans and French followed, with perfumes becoming the most sought-after gifts for royalty. The first synthetic perfume to gain mass attention was Chanel No. 5, when we were still unaware of the carcinogenic effect of the ingredients added to fragrance concoctions.

Natural perfumes are made from precious plant extracts and oils – ingredients that are way too expensive for the mainstream industry. If you think the perfume you bought on sale was a bargain, consider the fact that it probably cost between 50 cents and two dollars for the company to manufacture that bottle of chemicals.

I guarantee you, if you switch to a pure natural perfume or essential oil blend, you'll get more compliments. There's an abundance of beautiful and beneficial scents in nature: rose, jasmine and sandalwood are just a few.

You can make your own essential oil blends to match your taste, whether you prefer floral, fruity or woody scents. When using essential oils, it's recommended you dilute them with a plant oil at a ratio of 3:10 or weaker. Some skin types may be more sensitive to essential oils and may require different ratios of dilution.

If you're going to go natural with your skincare, then you should be doing the same thing with your make-up. Granted – there is no such thing as the perfect natural mascara (I admit I still use a conventional one sometimes), but everything else that touches my skin is natural. The fact is, if you removed all the artificial scents, preservatives, silicones and mineral oils from conventional make-up, you wouldn't have much product left. Natural make-up is infused with skin-loving botanicals, so you will likely notice a difference in your skin health just from changing your make-up. It took a little while for me to find the best brands, but there are some superb ones. (Feel free to get in touch with me to find out what they are!)

Travel beauty

If there is one thing that will force you into being creative, it's traveling. How can you decant a thick cream into a bottle under 100 ml (3.4 fl oz)? How do you fit an entire bathroom of cosmetics into a teeny-tiny case? I've picked up a few travel beauty hacks in my time. You learn to be extra savvy when you live in Australia, and a trip overseas means you'll be on a plane for approximately one billion hours (it's an exaggeration, but it can feel like it). I travel almost everywhere with only carry-on luggage, no matter where I'm going or for how long, so for me, it's all about being minimal and focused on what I need to lug around with me. Don't expect that you'll be able to give yourself the same care and attention that you do when you're at home – you just won't have the same amount of products on hand, and that's OK! You're on holidays, after all.

MY 10 TRAVEL BEAUTY TIPS AND TRICKS

1. Don't bother with nail polish or getting a manicure the day before you head off. Nobody likes chipped polish, and when it happens, you'll have to buy nail polish remover. Just keep your nails short and clean; all you'll need is a nail file and maybe a cuticle clipper.

2. A little roll-on bottle of your fragrance or an essential oil bottle is super easy to travel with. A woman in the bathroom pulling a giant bottle of perfume from her bag for a spritz will never cease to amaze me. How could she afford the space for it?

3. Antibacterial wipes are a must. Planes aren't the most hygienic of places. As soon as you get on, wipe down everything you're going to touch, including the tray and remote control.

4. Drink a ton of water, and infuse it with a fizzing multivitamin tablet. The nutrition you'll be getting on a plane is, to put it lightly, subpar. Vitamins will be your best friend on planes.

5. Rhodiola is an adaptogenic herb that's immune-boosting and available in capsule form. It's thought to also help protect you from radiation, which you'll be dousing yourself in, unbeknownst to you.

6. On the plane, I wouldn't bother with make-up. It is all about looking after your skin, which is about to be put through the wringer. You'll notice how dry your skin will get, so it's time to whip out a nourishing moisturiser. You'll want to start your day by using a body oil. Don't worry about fake tan either – this will dry out your skin even more. For your face, add an oil serum before your moisturiser, and apply an eye cream.

7. In your carry-on cosmetics case, you should have the following: hand sanitiser, face moisturiser, eye cream, face mist, lip balm and a sheet face mask if you like. Less is more! I'd also recommend a sunscreen or BB cream, as the UV you're exposed to on planes (if you're sitting by the window) can be strong.

8. Don't forget eye drops, or a silk eye mask for that matter.

9. Depending on the length of your flight, you might want to pack your own snacks. Aeroplane food is very salty and can increase your body's water retention. Keep walking on the flight, and if you can, get your legs elevated to avoid the dreaded puffy cankles at the end of your flight.

10. Shower as soon as you get to your destination. Exfoliate your body and wash your hair. (Dry brushing works wonders, page 85.) There's nothing like a shower after a long flight to make you feel like a newborn.

....

Tips & Tricks: When travelling, I always take earplugs (the ones they give you on the plane are rubbish), a few herbal tea sachets and a pair of disposable socks, which I wear all around the plane and throw away when the flight is over.

Jet lag

Jet lag isn't compulsory. The most effective method I have found is to try to reset your body clock the night before you leave by setting your watch to the time of your destination. Often, this means you'll be running low on sleep the day you fly out, but you'll probably sleep better on the plane. My sleep tips coming up on page 164 will also work on the plane. Some people swear by melatonin tablets. For me, a glass or two of red wine is just as good.

Meditating throughout the flight can help prevent jet lag, as can exercising when you land. Whatever you do, do not succumb to the 20-minute midday nap, or you'll find yourself waking up at 6 pm, ready to start your day.

....

Tips & Tricks: Contact lens cases can make the perfect little containers for small amounts of product to take on the plane.

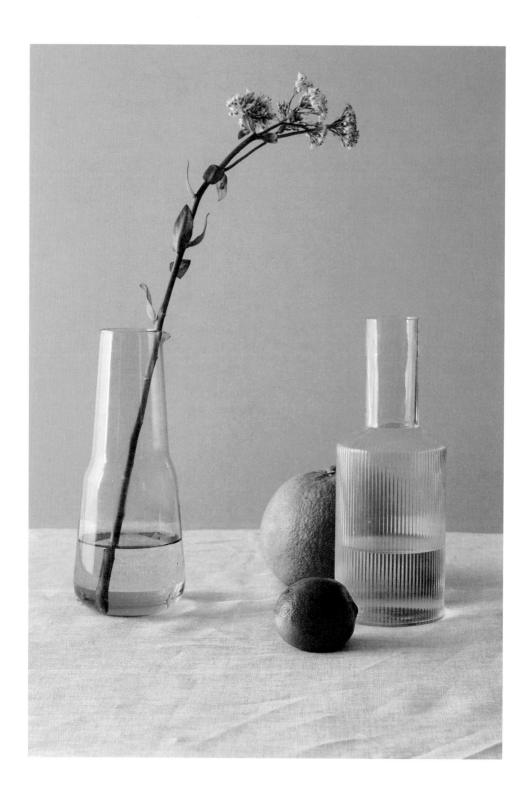

Nurturing your psychological environment

The connection between mind, body and spirit has been recognised throughout history. I believe we've been a little distracted and have wandered from taking this connection seriously, but I am seeing a swing back to reconnecting our physical selves with our mind and spirit. When we take care of our bodies, we need to take care of how we feel on the inside too. Both are acts of self-love.

There's a huge link between our psychology and our physical bodies. You've probably seen it yourself. I certainly have. Our physical health and beauty are inextricably tied to stress and our emotions. For example, anxiety can show up as rashes and lead to an accelerated ageing process.

During those times that I have been most stressed in my life, I've seen my skin lose its plumpness and become pale and dull. Wrinkles seem to sporadically pop up, not to mention the changes in my hair.

If I were to write all I could on emotional and spiritual wellbeing, it would have to be an entirely new book. Instead, I'll share the tools and techniques that I have tried myself. The thing to remember is, just like everyone's ability to cope with stressors is different, their release techniques will be different too.

Forget about trying to avoid stress your whole life. We all encounter stress and emotional adversity during our lives. Stress gives us the ability to get to know ourselves better. It can be what hurts us, but also what helps us. Resilience is tested, and so is our patience. When tough things happen, we pull out the lessons where we can and learn how to look after ourselves in the process.

....

Tips & Tricks: The practice of visualisation is incredibly powerful. It doesn't matter how far you are from where you'd like to be; take the time to visualise being where you want to be, and feel the emotion of that. When things are really bad, you may need to fake it 'til you make it. Or just put one foot in front of the other and keep going. After all, the only way out is through.

The best thing you can do for your stress, I believe, is to see things as they are, not worse than they are, like we tend to do. Thoughts can become more permanent, so try to steer your mind in the right direction. Reach for the low-hanging fruit of a better-feeling thought if you need to; you don't have to pretend that everything is awesome and wonderful when you feel like you're in the emotional trenches.

Sometimes, staying zen just isn't a possibility. I certainly have felt at times in my life that meditation and gratefulness just aren't options. Sometimes we just need to succumb to our feelings and let them infiltrate our bodies. When my mum had a series of heart attacks (she's fine now!), I cried every night for ten days. Then I began to pull myself together. I was also coping with a recently broken heart that made it really tough to even function. (I could write a whole book on heartbreak – true heartbreak will steal your senses. Food has no taste, colours are dull, and it's hard to see how people around you are still functioning so normally when you feel so disconnected.)

So let the feels come in. Let the pain in, allow it to teach you, but don't let it overstay its welcome. It's not easy to heal yourself, but it's the greatest lesson you'll ever learn, and you'll be able to empathise with others like never before.

Sleep it off

Sleep is crucial for your body and brain to repair at night, as well as for reducing stress. Insomnia has some very bad health effects: it's linked to wider waistlines because sleep deprivation reduces the levels of leptin, an appetite-suppressing hormone. Even chronic diseases like heart attacks and diabetes have been linked to sleep deprivation. If that's not enough to make you want to invest in a stable sleep pattern, then perhaps the physical attributes of sleeplessness will put you off, such as the increase in wrinkles and dry skin.

Tips & Tricks: Limit technology use at night! The blue light emitted from our devices keeps us awake.

To help with sleep, there are a few things you can try. You can use a diffuser to disperse essential oils such as chamomile, lavender and rose while you sleep. You can reach for foods naturally rich in melatonin, like cherries (these are by far the best food source of melatonin), rice and mustard seeds, and take supplements like high-grade magnesium and B vitamins, which are best

taken at night to assist sleep. Flower essences are also incredibly powerful for sleep (and for hangovers!). Candles are soothing; just be sure to blow them out before you fall asleep. I met a naturopath who swears by staring at a flame for a few minutes before bed to get the best night's sleep. It's worth a try! A traditional Chinese medicine trick for sleep is to dunk your feet in hot water for a few minutes before bed. It's thought that the water draws all the high energy out, leaving you much less energetic.

Tips & Tricks: Magnesium is best absorbed through your skin, so try to find it infused into body oils. It can make your skin itchy at first until you get used to it.

Exercise and earthing

The best remedy for stress and certainly for sleeplessness is, in my opinion, exercise. High-intensity exercise also helps you secrete human growth hormone (HGH), the miracle hormone that slows down our ageing. Beyond HGH and the rush of happy hormones we get from exercise, it importantly adds a good daily routine that we can rely on to help us stay sane and cope with what the day brings.

Beauty and exercise are my non-negotiables. If you can control nothing else in your day, you can control how you look after yourself. I like to try all different kinds of exercise, but I tend to stay away from group training sessions that include lots of weights, as I like to feel feminine with my exercise. I've got enough of a fighting mentality without working myself up at boxing! (At the moment, I'm into reformer Pilates and solo gym sessions.) If high-intensity exercise isn't your thing, then that's fine. A 20-minute walk can do wonders. No matter how bad I feel, if

I go for a walk I always come home feeling at least a fraction better than before I went out. It's good for our bodies, and it shifts our perspective and gets us out of our heads.

One of my aims in life is to reconnect humans with the natural world we have become separated from, so it will come as no surprise that I implore you to take off your shoes (and clothes if you legally can!), and get all touchy with nature. If you can, walk barefoot on some grass or the beach. This is called grounding or earthing. It's in age-old practices like shinrin-yoku, Japanese forest bathing. The idea is that direct physical contact with the vast supply of electrons on the surface of the earth contributes to physiological wellness. Emerging evidence shows that contact with the earth can be an effective strategy against inflammation, pain, chronic stress, poor sleep and even cardiovascular disease.

Meditation

The benefits of meditation are cumulative; meditation shouldn't only be used when you're having a crisis, even though it can make you feel instantly better. The roots of meditation have been traced all the way back to prehistoric times, although it wasn't until the 1960s and 1970s that it really began to influence Western culture.

When I was about twenty, I learned Vedic meditation. I haven't always practised as you should (20 minutes twice per day), but it's a practice that has stayed with me. There's nothing like the total transcendent feeling of this meditation.

Although I am biased towards a Vedic style of meditation, there are many other methods to try, and you can learn from taking classes and even through apps. If you're learning meditation (particularly Vedic style), you'll no doubt also be familiar with breathing techniques, which can have an instant calming effect.

I once went on a Vedic meditation and yoga weekend. In those three days, we spent nine hours per day completing cycles of a 40-minute yoga sequence, followed by a few minutes of alternate nostril breathing and then 20 minutes of meditation. I felt incredible after, but you can do a similar circuit at home.

Breath work

Breathing techniques are incredibly useful and there are countless versions. There are courses that teach you to breathe in certain ways that actually make you hallucinate or even pass out. I went to a class a few months ago, with around fifty other people, where we focused on a specific (difficult) breathing technique for about 20 minutes before someone in the room had an orgasm. Yep – breathing can be that powerful.

Box breathing is a much gentler technique I came across recently. It's simple but calming. Just breathe in for a count of four, hold for four, breathe out for four, hold for four, and repeat for at least four times.

Herbal treatments

Herbal treatments can help with stress, as can adaptogens, which you'll often see in stores (mostly online) in the form of mushrooms. (Don't worry – they're not psychoactive.) Adaptogens help bring your body and mind back to their balanced states. I have tried mushroom extract adaptogens and the herb rhodiola, which is known for its immune-boosting activities. Ashwagandha goes into my smoothie every day. It's an Ayurvedic herb that is known for its stress-relieving benefits, and I have found it works really well.

Tips & Tricks: When all else fails, there are prescription drugs to assist you in dealing with your anxiety or depression. They can be absolute lifesavers when appropriately prescribed, and can give you just that bit of support whilst you heal yourself.

Alternative therapies

If I am feeling out of whack and really need to ground myself, I find that alternative healing therapies really help. Reiki is a beautiful practice (I'm trained in it myself), and so is kinesiology and many other energy-based practices. I occasionally see a chiropractor who focuses on using breath to heal energy blocks and therefore aches and pain in the body. Throughout many ancient healing modalities, it's thought that our bodies store unprocessed emotion, leading to pain, which can become disease.

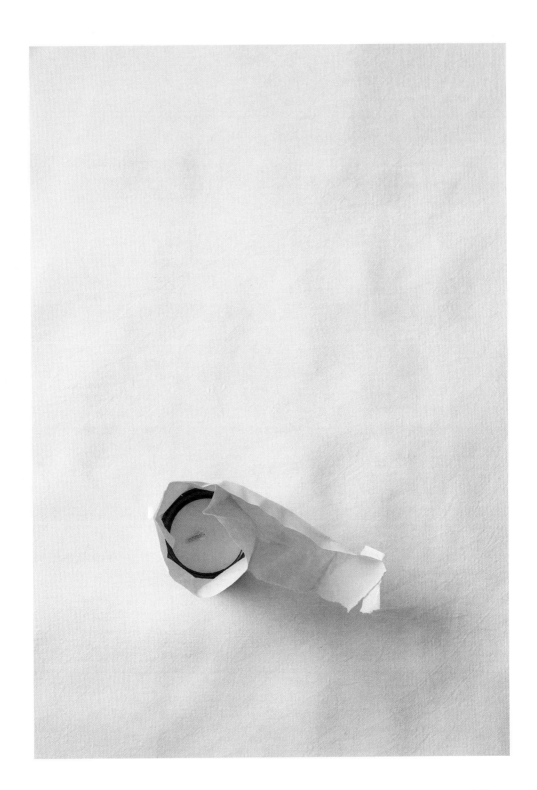

Outro

So, where to from here?

You'll know now that you are responsible for your own beauty and wellness. What a sense of control and power that gives you! I'm hoping by now you've incorporated at least some of the natural beauty and wellness rituals in this book into your life.

What I don't want you to do is stress about overhauling your lifestyle. If you want to live like I do – treating your body much like a natural beauty and wellness guinea pig, and being mildly obsessive about it – then go for it. Remember that there is nothing wrong with satisfying your somewhat pleasure-seeking behaviours every now and then. Too much restriction on your wants and cravings breeds stress, and that's the worst thing for our beauty and wellness. If I want a cocktail or some chocolate, I'm having it. Those close to me would know better than to suggest otherwise. If you're not living your best 100 per cent natural lifestyle because you can't let go of your favourite conventional lipstick, it's not the end of the world!

Give yourself time. You wouldn't expect freshly planted seeds to bloom the very next day. Give yourself time to adjust and the results will come at the right time, some quicker than others – some physical, some emotional. Growth and progress are all we need to feel. Lasting transformation does take work, especially when we are focusing on wellness as a whole, rather than just the way we look.

Beauty practices aren't just about physically looking our best; the most beautiful thing you'll find with the natural beauty rituals is the connection you cultivate with yourself and with nature. You'll become aware of how you may have been so distracted by daily life that you forgot how to be present. The meditative nature of self-care practices and the natural progression of self-love will be a gift that keeps on giving throughout your life, to both yourself and to those around you.

Wellness is a commitment, not a fling. Be curious, experiment, be creative and, most importantly, have fun.

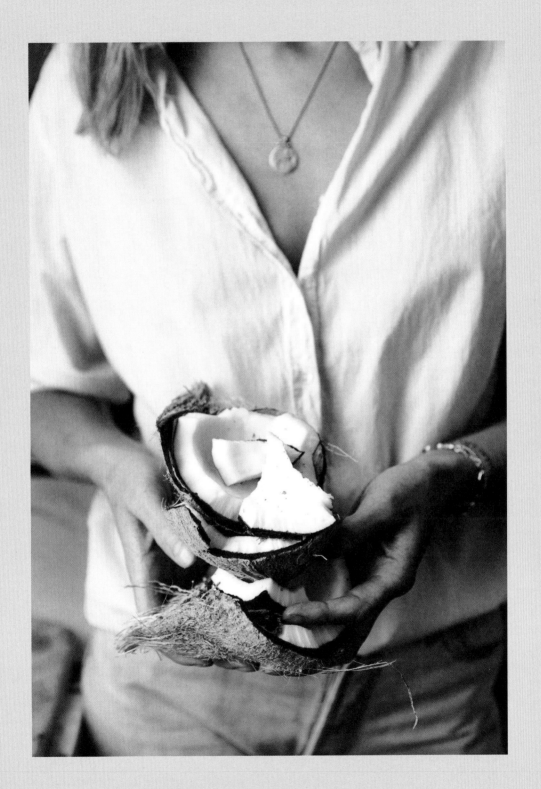

Index

sesame 137
   sweet almond 19, 63, 77, 103,
      104, 106, 114, 123, 142
   tamanu 22, 25
   tea tree 23, 24, 27, 139
omega-3 fatty acids 18, 19, 128,
   147, 150
omega-9 fatty acids 19
orange 91

P

papain 38, 41
papaya 41
parabens 13, 80, 156
perfume 30, 117
   natural 159
petrochemicals 155–6
pH levels 25, 46, 94, 116, 147
phthalates 155
pimples 23, 152
pineapple 41
prebiotics 10, 48
probiotics 10, 152
product labels 155–6
protein 146

R

reiki 167
resveratrol 10, 41
retinoids 24, 25, 38, 53
   retinol 22, 24, 25, 43, 53
   retinyl palmitate 53
rhassoul mud 28, 90
rice
   milk 147
   water 32
rice bran
   powder 29
   wax 109
rosacea 29, 32, 54
rosemary 129, 132
rose petals 89, 93, 98, 118
rosewater 35, 41, 117
routine 10
   acne-prone skin 25
   dry skin 22
   oily skin 25
   mature skin 43
   sensitive skin 32
rutin 29

S

salmon 18
salt 23, 75, 77, 90, 93, 123

saltwater 23
scalp 129, 136
   cleanser 137
   massage 135
   serum 137
   treatment 135
scrubs 47, 74–7, 81, 85, 123, 147
sea salt 23, 134
seaweed 18, 75
seeds
   hemp 18
   chia 18
serum 10, 19, 22, 25, 32, 43, 54,
   67, 137
shea butter 44, 98, 109, 111, 112,
   117, 142
silica 128
skincare 10, 16–51, 73–98,
   120–3, 152, 159, 160
   skin types 16–51
sleep 164
solvents 140, 155
steam treatment 17, 32, 43, 69, 70
sterolin 19
stress 163
stretch marks 81
sugar 47, 76, 82
sun
   care 120–1
   damage 38, 69–70, 120–1
   screens 120–1
   rescue spray 123
sunflower wax 109

T

tea 69, 80
   black 104
   brahmi 69
   burdock 80
   calendula 70, 94
   chai 104
   chamomile 70, 94
   dandelion 60, 80
   gotu kola 69
   green 42, 59, 60–1, 67, 69–70,
   herbal 69–70
   jasmine 91
   matcha powder 75, 90, 91
   nettle 80
   peppermint 59
   rooibos 69
   sage 70
   white 42, 69, 91
tequila 77

toner 27, 41
tongue scraping 10
toxic ingredients 8, 13, 38, 62,
   67, 101, 109, 116, 117, 120, 127,
   134, 140
travel tips 160–1
   jet lag 161
turmeric 29, 36, 42

V

vanilla bean 76, 90, 98, 104, 106
Vedic meditation 11, 165
vegetables 42, 61, 147
vitamin A 19, 38, 39, 42, 53,
   101, 139, 147, 150
vitamin B 54, 61, 139
   B7 128
vitamin C 10, 19, 22, 25, 29, 38,
   39, 42, 43, 53, 54, 101, 104,
   123, 147, 151
vitamin D 103, 121, 150
vitamin E 42, 43, 63, 67, 90,
   103, 104, 123, 136, 142
vitamin K 25, 32

W

wakame 18
walnuts 150
water 31, 80, 148
waxes 101, 109
wine 41
witch hazel 17, 24, 123

Y

yoghurt 51

Z

zinc 30, 32, 121, 139, 151

Recipes

Thank You

They say everyone comes into your life for a season or for a reason, and I can say I am a lucky little dumpling to have had so many life-changing teachers in my life, all around the world.

To the beautiful team at Hardie Grant Publishing, who I *still* can't believe took a chance on me. You are dream makers.

My friends. I often think of how lucky I am to have such a special relationship with you all. Just couldn't do life without you all. Thank you for laughing with me whilst I go on about the newest superfood powder and the cycles of the moon.

The true loves of my life, for pushing me to exactly where I needed to go. Even when it really hurt.

My parents. Thank you for never telling me to choose the less risky option and never questioning me when I decided to fly to the other side of the world.

Mum, for devoting your life to us kids and for being the most selfless person I will ever know.

Dad, for instilling in me the importance of playfulness, a love for the natural world and for seeing what you want and just going for it.

Everybody who has walked with me and helped me grow in my life journey so far, and those who will walk with me in the future. From my meditation teachers, my naturopaths, my Vedic wisdom–filled friends and every single person who supports my business and mission to reduce the separation between humans and nature.

I hope I can give back to the world all the good energy, love and growth I have been blessed with.

About Maddy

Maddy Daisy Dixon lives by the motto that beauty is wellness and wellness is beauty. This applies to every aspect of her life, from the food she eats and the way she lives to the beauty products and rituals she incorporates into her life.

After travelling the world and working in the fashion industry, Maddy has seen beauty from all angles. Her beauty ethos is to find the most effective natural ingredients and treatments to enhance our natural beauty, create rituals of self-care and get us all closer to nature.

Maddy is the founder of two natural beauty businesses, Flora Remedia and Wildwish.

You can keep in touch with her on Instagram: **@maddy.daisy**

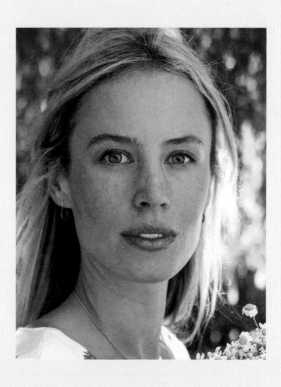

Published in 2020 by Hardie Grant Books, an imprint of Hardie Grant Publishing

Hardie Grant Books (Melbourne)
Building 1, 658 Church Street
Richmond, Victoria 3121

Hardie Grant Books (London)
5th & 6th Floors
52–54 Southwark Street
London SE1 1UN

hardiegrantbooks.com

A catalogue record for this
book is available from the
National Library of Australia

Botanical Beauty Hunter
ISBN 978 1 74379 642 9

10 9 8 7 6 5 4 3 2 1

Publishing Director: Pam Brewster
Project Editor: Joanna Wong
Editor: Allison Hiew
Photographer: Armelle Habib
Stylist: Lee Blaylock
Design Manager: Jessica Lowe
Designer: Murray Batten
Production Manager: Todd Rechner
Production Coordinator: Mietta Yans

Colour reproduction by Splitting Image Colour Studio
Printed in China by Leo Paper Products LTD.

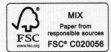